When Therapists Cry

When Therapists Cry addresses one of the most authentic and singularly human experiences a therapist can have in therapy: crying. While therapist crying in therapy is the explicit focus of this book, it is used as a springboard for understanding the various ways in which therapists' emotions come alive—and become visible—in the therapy room. In depth clinical examples and conceptualizations from expert contributors illustrate what the experience of therapist crying looks and feels like: why therapists cry, how crying impacts the therapist and the treatment, what therapists feel about their tears, and the many ways in which therapists may engage with their own tears in order to facilitate therapeutic progress, ensure appropriate professional conduct, and deepen their clinical work.

Amy Blume-Marcovici, PsyD, has published numerous articles on topics ranging from psychological testing to clinical work with dreams. Her research focuses on process-oriented and relational aspects of psychotherapy, particularly therapists' emotional expressions in therapy. She is on the editorial board of the journal *Psychotherapy*.

"Since modern studies of adult emotional crying began in the 1980s, there has been a veritable explosion of research on the subject. Until the publication of *When Therapists Cry*, however, one of the relatively unexplored aspects of the phenomenon of emotional crying has been the dynamics of crying in the context of psychotherapy. Amy Blume-Marcovici and her collaborators in this important new book have now remedied this situation, expanding and enriching our understanding of crying and therapy enormously."

—**Randolph R. Cornelius, PhD,** professor of psychological science, Vassar College, and coeditor (with Ad Vingerhoets) of *Adult Crying: A Biopsychosocial Approach*

"In this much-needed volume, Dr. Blume-Marcovici and her colleagues provide a vital forum for a long neglected topic in a beautifully rendered discussion of what happens when therapists are moved to tears. Each of the chapters is thoughtful, meaningful, and inspiring. This will be a most useful book for clinicians of all persuasions and all levels of training."

—**Steve Tuber, PhD, ABPP,** professor of psychology and director of clinical training, City College of New York

"*When Therapists Cry* is a long awaited resource that offers valuable insight and wisdom into crying and feeling in the therapy room. This is not only about knowing another but also having awareness about being known. It will help you figure out how your honest presence can promote positive change and healing. You will read and reread this book and it will empower you as a therapist. A real treasure that can open new possibilities!"

—**Rosemary B. Mennuti, EdD,** retired professor of school psychology, Philadelphia College of Osteopathic Medicine

"Therapists' tears are often seen as embarrassing, intrusive, and even a shameful breach of convention and technique. This thoughtful collection of research findings and personal consulting room experiences helps us see that these moments of humanity may in fact lead to deeper relationships and even a therapeutic turning point. Teachers and students will find a lot to think about here, and so will others who want to learn more about therapy itself."

—**Ann Shearer,** author of *Why Don't Psychotherapists Laugh? Enjoyment and the Consulting Room*

When *Therapists* Cry

REFLECTIONS ON THERAPISTS' TEARS IN THERAPY

EDITED BY

AMY BLUME-MARCOVICI

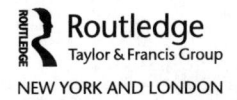

Routledge
Taylor & Francis Group
NEW YORK AND LONDON

First published 2017
by Routledge
711 Third Avenue, New York, NY 10017

and by Routledge
2 Park Square, Milton Park, Abingdon, Oxon OX14 4RN

Routledge is an imprint of the Taylor & Francis Group, an informa business

© 2017 Amy Blume-Marcovici

The right of Amy Blume-Marcovici to be identified as the author of the editorial material, and of the authors for their individual chapters, has been asserted in accordance with sections 77 and 78 of the Copyright, Designs and Patents Act 1988.

All rights reserved. No part of this book may be reprinted or reproduced or utilized in any form or by any electronic, mechanical, or other means, now known or hereafter invented, including photocopying and recording, or in any information storage or retrieval system, without permission in writing from the publishers.

Trademark notice: Product or corporate names may be trademarks or registered trademarks, and are used only for identification and explanation without intent to infringe.

Library of Congress Cataloging in Publication Data
Names: Blume-Marcovici, Amy, editor.
Title: When therapists cry : reflections on therapists' tears in therapy / edited by Amy Blume-Marcovici.
Description: New York, NY : Routledge, Taylor & Francis Group, 2017. | Includes bibliographical references and indexes.
Identifiers: LCCN 2016044541| ISBN 9781138927308 (hbk) | ISBN 9781138927315 (pbk.) | ISBN 9781315673059 (ebk)
Subjects: | MESH: Psychotherapy | Crying—psychology | Psychotherapeutic Processes | Empathy | Professional–Patient Relations | Attitude of Health Personnel
Classification: LCC RC480.5 | NLM WM 420 | DDC 616.89/14—dc23
LC record available at https://lccn.loc.gov/2016044541

ISBN: 978-1-138-92730-8 (hbk)
ISBN: 978-1-138-92731-5 (pbk)
ISBN: 978-1-315-67305-9 (ebk)

Typeset in Garamond
by Swales & Willis Ltd, Exeter, Devon, UK

In memory of my mother, Joan H. Blume, a dedicated therapist and loving mom.

CONTENTS

About the Editor ix
List of Contributors xi
Acknowledgments xvii

Amy Blume-Marcovici, Introduction 1

PART I: THE TRACKS OF OUR TEARS: AN ORIENTATION TO CRYING

1 *Lauren M. Bylsma, Asmir Gračanin, and Ad J. J. M. Vingerhoets*, Why Humans Weep 7

2 *Amy Blume-Marcovici, Ronald A. Stolberg, Mojgan Khademi, Anthony Mackie, and Catelijne 't Lam*, Tracking Our Tears: Research on Therapist Crying in Therapy 23

PART II: CONSTRUCTS OF CRYING: UNDERSTANDING TEARS THROUGH THEORY

3 *Judith Kay Nelson*, The Feeling Is Mutual: Therapist Crying From an Attachment/Caregiving Perspective 43

4 *Andrea Bloomgarden*, An Eye-Opening Eye Infection: Treating Therapists' Tears as Self-Disclosure 59

5 *Mark J. Hilsenroth, Jason Mayotte-Blum, Klara Kuutmann, and Kristen L. Capps Umphlet*, Therapeutic Immediacy: If Your Tears Could Speak, What Would They Say? 73

CONTENTS

6 *Patricia Harney*, The Psychoanalyst's Tears: From Abstinence to Authenticity   89

7 *Dennis Tirch and Laura R. Silberstein*, Hearing the Cries of the World: The Role of Therapists' Tears in Compassion-Focused Therapy   101

8 *Paul McGinley*, Existential Therapy and the Transformative Possibilities of Therapists' Tears   115

PART III: THE CLIENTS WITH WHOM WE CRY

9 *Maxine Harris*, The Tears of Abuse   131

10 *Eleanor F. Counselman*, Tears and the Dying Client   143

11 *Fredric E. Rabinowitz*, Entering the No-Cry Zone: Men and the Chords of Connection   155

12 *Jerrold R. Brandell*, M. Night Shyamalan's *The Sixth Sense*: Relational Authenticity, Self-Disclosure, and a Child Therapist's Tears   165

13 *Wendy N. Davis*, Tears of the Emerging Parent: Therapists' Tears in Working With Pregnant and Postpartum Clients   183

14 *Amy Blume-Marcovici, Kelsey E. Schraufnagel, Mojgan Khademi, and Ronald A. Stolberg*, Supervising Our Tears: A Guide for Supervisors and Trainees   199

Index   219

ABOUT THE EDITOR

Amy Blume-Marcovici, PsyD, received her master's degree in Psychology from Teachers College, Columbia University, and her doctorate in clinical psychology from Alliant International University in San Diego. She received clinical training at the University of California San Diego (UCSD) and the UCSD Center for Mindfulness, San Diego State University, and Cambridge Health Alliance/Harvard Medical School. She has published numerous articles on topics ranging from psychological testing to clinical work with dreams. Her research focuses on process-oriented and relational aspects of psychotherapy and particularly therapists' emotional expressions in therapy. She is on the editorial board of the journal *Psychotherapy*. She lives and works in Portland, Oregon.

CONTRIBUTORS

Andrea Bloomgarden, PhD, is a clinical psychologist with a psychotherapy practice at Bloomgarden, Ostroff & Associates in Philadelphia. She is co-editor of the book *Psychotherapist Revealed: Therapists Speak About Self-Disclosure in Psychotherapy*. She speaks and writes about therapist authenticity and self-disclosure.

Jerrold R. Brandell, PhD, is distinguished professor and coordinator, Doctoral Concentration in Clinical Scholarship, Wayne State University School of Social Work (Detroit, MI). He is (founding) editor-in-chief of *Psychoanalytic Social Work*, and author/editor of 12 books and more than 50 articles, book chapters, and other publications. Recognized as a distinguished practitioner by the National Academies of Practice in 2001, he maintains a part-time practice in psychoanalysis and psychotherapy in Ann Arbor, MI.

Lauren M. Bylsma, PhD, is an assistant professor at the University of Pittsburgh Department of Psychiatry. Her research focuses on understanding emotional functioning in depressed individuals. Her work on crying has focused on relationships between crying and mood, as well as the influence of individual differences, context, and interpersonal factors on crying behavior and its effects. She is the author of numerous articles and book chapters.

Kristen L. Capps Umphlet, PhD, received her doctorate in clinical psychology from Adelphi University. She works at The Lourie Center for Children's Social and Emotional Wellness, where she specializes in therapy with young children and their families, particularly around issues of trauma. Dr. Capps' research interests include psychotherapy process and outcome, intervention studies, and strengthening the relationship between research and clinical practice.

LIST OF CONTRIBUTORS

Eleanor F. Counselman, EdD, ABPP, CGP, LFAGPA, is a psychologist with an adult psychotherapy practice of individuals, couples, and groups in Belmont, MA. She is board-certified in counseling psychology by the American Board of Professional Psychology, is a certified group psychotherapist, and is trained in emotionally focused therapy for couples. She is the President of the American Group Psychotherapy Association and was on the faculty of the Harvard Medical School for 25 years. She has published extensively on individual, couple, and group therapy, and psychotherapy supervision.

Wendy N. Davis, PhD, has a counseling and consulting practice in Portland, OR, specializing in depression, anxiety, creativity, and communication, with a special focus on pregnancy and postpartum mental health. She is the Executive Director for Postpartum Support International. She is the founding director of Oregon's Baby Blues Connection parent support organization, and serves as its clinical advisor and volunteer training consultant. Wendy is a certified perinatal mood and anxiety disorders trainer and conducts international trainings and consultations and gives keynote addresses on perinatal mental health.

Asmir Gračanin, PhD, is a senior research assistant in the Department of Psychology at the University of Rijeka, Croatia. His research interests comprise emotion and personality, especially their evolutionary origins and physiological aspects. His research on crying focuses on biological functions of crying, signal value, and effects on well-being.

Patricia Harney, PhD, is Interim Acting Chief of Psychology and Director of Psychology Internship Training at the Cambridge Health Alliance/Harvard Medical School. She maintains a practice in psychotherapy and psychoanalysis in Cambridge, MA. She received her Certificate in Psychoanalysis from the Massachusetts Institute of Psychoanalysis. Dr. Harney has presented and published professional articles on topics related to trauma, supervision, and clinical development.

Maxine Harris, PhD, is the co-founder and CEO of Community Connections, a behavioral health and residential service provider in the District of Columbia. She is the author of several books on trauma, early loss, and clinical case management. Dr. Harris has also served as the principal investigator on local and federal grants concerning issues of trauma, substance addiction, HIV, and homelessness. She is currently working on a book on trauma-informed care.

LIST OF CONTRIBUTORS

Mark J. Hilsenroth, PhD, ABAP, is a professor of psychology at the Derner Institute of Advanced Psychological Studies at Adelphi University and the primary investigator of the Adelphi University Psychotherapy Project. He is currently editor of the American Psychological Association Division 29 journal *Psychotherapy*. His areas of professional interest include personality assessment, training/supervision, psychotherapy process, and treatment outcomes.

Mojgan Khademi, PsyD, is a clinical psychologist, psychoanalyst, and associate professor at Alliant International University in San Diego, CA. She was the 2014 recipient of the American Psychoanalytic Association's Edith Sabshin Teaching Award. She is the director and clinical supervisor at the Center for Applied Psychology and Services, which provides low-cost mental health services to the San Diego community.

Klara Kuutmann, MS, received a master of science in psychology from Uppsala University, Sweden. Currently she works as a clinical psychologist at a psychiatric inpatient clinic at the hospital of Falun, Dalarna, Sweden. Her research interests include therapeutic immediacy as an intervention in therapy and psychotherapy treatments for panic disorder, as well as "common factors" in psychotherapy.

Anthony Mackie, PsyD, is a clinical psychologist in private practice in Melbourne, Australia. His research interests include attachment theory, emotion theory, and mechanisms of change in psychotherapy.

Jason Mayotte-Blum, PhD, is a licensed clinical psychologist working in university mental health, while maintaining a private practice. He received a Masters in Clinical Psychology from Pepperdine University, and a doctorate in Clinical Psychology from Adelphi University. He completed his internship and postdoctoral training at Emory University. His research interests include psychotherapy process and outcome, therapeutic immediacy, couples therapy, and addiction treatment.

Paul McGinley, PhD, ADEP, is an existential psychotherapist in private practice and lecturer in existential-phenomenological psychotherapy at Regent's University, London, where he researches into the phenomenology of crying. He was Chair of the Society for Existential Analysis for six years and is an active member of the UK Council for Psychotherapy.

Judith Kay Nelson, MSW, PhD, is the former Dean and currently on the faculty of the Sanville Institute for Clinical Social Work and Psychotherapy. She has taught and presented throughout the United States and Europe on topics related to crying, grief, laughter, and attachment and is the author of *Seeing Through Tears: Crying and Attachment* (Brunner-Routledge, 2005), *What Made Freud Laugh: An Attachment Perspective on Laughter* (Routledge, 2012), co-editor of *Adult Attachment in Clinical Social Work* (Springer, 2010), and author of numerous articles and chapters on laughter, crying, grief, and attachment.

Fredric E. Rabinowitz, PhD, has been a professor of psychology at the University of Redlands since 1984. Since that time he has maintained a private practice specializing in working with men in therapy. Dr. Rabinowitz has authored and co-authored numerous articles and four books. He is a fellow of the American Psychological Association and the past president of the Society for the Psychological Study of Men and Masculinity, a division of the American Psychological Association.

Kelsey E. Schraufnagel, PsyD, is a licensed psychologist in San Francisco, CA. She specializes in providing evidence-based treatment for anxiety and chronic and recurrent mood disorders at Gateway Psychiatric Services. Dr. Schraufnagel earned her doctorate in clinical psychology from Alliant International University in San Diego. She completed a predoctoral internship at University of Colorado-Boulder's Wardenburg Health Center and her postdoctoral training at the Center for Anxiety and Emotion Regulation Disorders and Gateway Psychiatric Services.

Laura R. Silberstein, PsyD, is the associate director of the Center for Compassion-Focused Therapy in New York. Dr. Silberstein also serves as adjunct assistant professor and consultant at Albert Einstein Medical College. She is the co-author of three books. Dr. Silberstein completed a two-year externship at the American Institute for Cognitive Therapy, in Manhattan, a predoctoral internship at Wyoming State Hospital, and a two-year postdoctoral fellowship in cognitive behavioral therapy at the Cognitive Behavioral Institute of Albuquerque, NM. Dr. Silberstein serves as a consultant and trainer in a range of third-generation behavior therapies, including compassion-focused therapy, acceptance and commitment therapy, and dialectical behavior therapy.

LIST OF CONTRIBUTORS

Ronald A. Stolberg, PhD, is a licensed clinical psychologist with an emphasis in child and family therapy. As an associate professor at Alliant International University, he teaches a variety of doctoral-level courses including those focused on psychological assessment and the development of clinical skills. He is author of numerous articles and several books, and is co-author of the award-winning book, *Teaching Kids to Think: Raising Confident, Thoughtful, and Independent Children in an Age of Instant Gratification* (Sourcebooks, 2015).

Catelijne 't Lam, MA, is a psychologist in the Netherlands working with adults at the community mental health agency, AmaCura. Her research focuses on emotions in therapy.

Dennis Tirch, PhD, is the founder and director of the Center for Compassion-Focused Therapy in New York and president of the Compassionate Mind Foundation USA. Dr. Tirch is the author of six books, and numerous chapters and peer-reviewed articles. He has served on the faculty of Cornell Weill Medical College and Albert Einstein Medical School. Dr. Tirch regularly conducts compassion-focused acceptance and commitment therapy and compassion-focused therapy trainings and workshops globally. He is a diplomate, fellow, and certified consultant and trainer for the Academy of Cognitive Therapy, founding fellow and president of the New York City Cognitive Behavioral Therapy Association, and founding president emeritus of the New York City chapter of the Association for Contextual Behavioral Science. Dr. Tirch is associate editor of the *Journal of Contextual Behavioral Therapy*.

Ad J. J. M. Vingerhoets, PhD, is a professor in the Department of Medical and Clinical Psychology at Tilburg University, the Netherlands. His expertise is on stress, emotions, and quality of life. His research on crying, nostalgia, homesickness, and "leisure sickness" has received much attention from the (inter)national media. He has published more than 300 articles and written 19 books.

ACKNOWLEDGMENTS

First and foremost, I want to thank the clients who have given me—and all of those who have contributed to this book—the privilege of experiencing the kind of connection that makes the therapy relationship, and indeed all human relationships, deeply gratifying; the kind of connection that can elicit tears.

A warm and awe-filled thank you to the esteemed clinicians who have contributed chapters to this book. It is your expertise, courage, shrewd intellect, compassion, and spirit that breathed life into this project. Thanks to the colleagues and mentors who have supported me in working on this book, and the related professional endeavors that led to it: Roland Stolberg, Mojgan Khademi, Patricia Harney, Chris Germer, Adam Conklin, Steve Hickman, Barry Farber, Carrie Sakai and the San Diego State University Counseling and Psychological Services staff, Neil Ribner, Donald Viglione, M. Bruce Stubbs, Paola Michelle Contreras, Ronald Del Castillo, Jessie Fontanella, Miriam Frankel, Elizabeth Freidin Baumann, Johanna Malaga, and Jacqui Sperling. Thanks in particular to my colleague and dear friend, Kelsey Schraufnagel, whose ever-ready wisdom, keen clinical insights, and humor have been invaluable to me.

Thank you to Anna Moore at Routledge who has been indispensable in the creation of this book from inception to publication. I appreciate your many insights and conscientiousness through our work together. Many thanks to all of the others at Routledge for their support, knowledge, and admirable creativity.

My profoundest gratitude to my family and friends. To my husband especially, for your love, your encouragement, and always believing in me. Without you, this book would not have happened. To my sister, for being my best friend and my own best editor. To my parents, for parenting me with love. And to my children, the lights of my life, who have taught me the true meaning of "tears of joy."

INTRODUCTION

Amy Blume-Marcovici

I could say that I became interested in the topic of therapists' tears in therapy during my graduate-school training, but the truth is, the topic of therapists' tears in therapy became interested in me. As I describe in a case example in Chapter 14 of this volume, I experienced tearing up with a client during my second year as a psychology trainee. When I reached out for supervision, my peers were fascinated by the subject of therapists' tears. I was even more intrigued to learn that many of my supervisors and teachers had never discussed the topic in all of their time in the profession. Opinions on the matter ranged widely—and passionately—but, regardless of stance on whether or not a therapist *should* ever tear up or cry in therapy, most everyone agreed that the topic of therapists' emotional expressions in therapy, and especially therapists' tears, should be addressed explicitly and openly.

After countless discussions with colleagues, therapists' tears—albeit captivating in and of themselves—became a symbol to me, a rich way to segue into conversation about mutuality and intersubjectivity in psychotherapy. When we cry—in therapy or otherwise—we are invoking our earliest form of communication: our bodies are reaching out to others, the physical distance between ourselves and others lessens, we allow ourselves to be deeply moved. In this way, therapists' tears, at their core, are about our *humanity* as psychotherapists. By focusing on therapists' tears as a discrete entity, I found that I could "operationalize" this otherwise quite incalculable topic. Thus I went on to explore therapists' tears in multiple research projects.

My first study on therapists' tears was an online survey, for which I offered $2 donations to a non-profit organization on behalf of each participant. I received over 700 responses so quickly, I had to close the study—I couldn't afford to keep going! My research participants often commented that they had never disclosed their experience of tears in therapy to anyone, but that these tears were deeply meaningful, an example of a sort of essential ingredient to the amorphic recipe of, as one respondent put it, a "strong therapeutic alliance." Alternatively, a smaller cohort of respondents described worry that their tears caused a rupture in the alliance and were a source of shame. After publishing several articles and conducting an interview with the BBC World Service's *Health Check* international news program on the topic of tears in therapy, I received many more emails from therapists and clients alike from around the world interested in what I had learned about therapists' tears.

So what had I learned? That this is a topic that people find compelling. What else had I learned? That the taboo around crying in our culture applies to the psychotherapy setting as well, a setting in which intense emotional work is often expected to lead to tears by the client, but tears of the therapist are sequestered in mystery and secrecy. Crying, it seems, is truly one of our most vulnerable behaviors, as therapists and as humans. It rarely feels fully in our control. It is a time when our body reveals our inner world to those outside of us, whether we want it to or not. There is vulnerability, shame, fascination, curiosity, repulsion, discomfort, and intrigue wrapped up in our cultural understanding of tears, and likewise in the topic of therapists' tears in therapy. Do therapists cry in therapy? Is there ever a place for therapist tears in the therapy room? To the former question, the answer is yes. Most therapists, although relatively infrequently, do tear up or cry in therapy at some point in their career. The answer to the second question is one I hope readers will answer for themselves after having read through the chapters in this book and, thus, having had the chance to reflect deeply on theoretical constructs that help us understand therapists' tears.

The book is divided into three parts. The first part, The Tracks of Our Tears: An Orientation to Crying (Chapters 1 and 2) provides an overview of what exactly crying is, and how it manifests in the therapy room. Outlining our understanding of crying in general and therapist crying in therapy specifically, these first chapters focus on the current state of research on crying. The chapters in the following two parts use clinical vignettes to illustrate a theme related to therapists' tears. Specifically, the second part, Constructs of Crying: Understanding Tears Through Theory (Chapters 3–8), explores various lenses through which we may understand therapists' tears. Each chapter provides an orientation to its "lens" (i.e., the lens of attachment, therapeutic immediacy, or a specific theoretical orientation) and then describes the way in which this lens helps us to understand therapist crying. The third part, The Clients With Whom We Cry (Chapters 9–14), focuses on the clinical significance of a clinician's tears in working with a specific client population: the ways in which a therapist may be provoked to tears in working with these specific client groups, and the potential positive impact and/or pitfalls of therapists' tears with these varying populations. In addition, clinical supervision and training on the topic of therapists' tears are addressed in this section.

This book is meant for clinicians at all levels of experience. Each chapter provides an overview of its specific topic—self-disclosure, compassion, trauma, child psychotherapy—and in this way provides a broad foundation of knowledge for a new clinician. Each chapter also delves deeply into the meaning and role of tears in therapy, a topic which therapists report often goes undiscussed in all of their training. Thus, experienced clinicians, who may have long had their own ideas about clients' and therapists' tears in therapy but never had the opportunity to discuss them, will have the chance to engage with such ideas in an organized framework for the first time. In addition, because tearing up as a therapist is a shared experience among therapists, it is my hope that this book will be useful for clinicians of all theoretical backgrounds and as such includes authors from varying theoretical orientations and presents transtheoretical concepts related to therapist tears.

While the vision for this book began as a series of ponderings on therapists' tears in therapy—an effort to give voice to the silence in our field surrounding the topic—thanks to the wise and empathic psychotherapists who have shared their stories and vast clinical knowledge in these chapters, it has grown into a reflection on the role of humanity and connection in psychotherapy. My hope for the reader is that this book will foster not only curiosity about tears in therapy—your own and your clients'—but reflection on the very nature of connection, attachment, caregiving, authenticity, intersubjectivity, disclosure, and mechanisms of change in our unique and most intimate of professions: helping people heal and grow.

THE TRACKS OF OUR TEARS: AN ORIENTATION TO CRYING

CHAPTER 1

WHY HUMANS WEEP

Lauren M. Bylsma, Asmir Gračanin, and Ad J. J. M. Vingerhoets

The capacity for shedding emotional tears is uniquely human, and this ubiquitous behavior, displayed from cradle to deathbed, is observed in all human societies across time (Provine, 2012; Trimble, 2012; Vingerhoets, 2013). In scientific terms, emotional crying is defined as the shedding of tears from the lacrimal apparatus in the absence of irritation of the eyes, often accompanied by facial muscle alterations, vocalizations, and sobbing (Patel, 1993). In one of the earliest known written accounts on tears, the ancient Roman poet Ovid (43 B.C.–A.D. 17) was known to have said, "It is some relief to weep; grief is satisfied and carried off by tears." Ovid additionally recommended lovers to show their tears to their beloved to convince them of the sincerity of their love, suggesting that tears can serve an important social function as well. It seems as if this poet was ahead of his time with respect to his understanding of the functions of tears. Although we all have experience with crying and scholars have speculated on its role throughout history, the specific functions of human emotional tears remain quite elusive. Recent theoretical developments and empirical findings allow us to reach some initial understanding of this, until now, poorly understood human behavior.

In the present chapter, we provide an overview of what is currently known about human emotional crying. We begin with evolutionary and developmental considerations. Next, we consider antecedents of adult crying and how they differ across individuals. This is followed by a discussion of the main functions of tears and empirical findings on their intraindividual and interindividual effects. We also consider the relationship of crying with mental and physical health. We conclude by describing the limited available research on crying in the therapy context, which will set the stage for the remainder of this volume focused on (therapists') tears in therapy.[1]

EVOLUTIONARY ORIGINS OF HUMAN EMOTIONAL CRYING

While many are familiar with Charles Darwin and his theory of evolution, it is less known that he also discussed human tears in his seminal work, *The Expression of the Emotions in Man and Animals* (1872). Darwin observed a connection between emotional tears and suffering, as well as between tears and tender feelings, and briefly addressed questions such as whether animals weep, developmental and cross-cultural aspects of crying, and frequent crying as a characteristic of melancholia. Disappointingly, however, he did not speculate on the potential evolutionary function of emotional tears. More recent theories have proposed that human emotional crying has its evolutionary origins in the acoustical signals mammals display when separated from their mother (Hasson, 2009; Murube, 2009; Provine, 2012; Trimble, 2012; Vingerhoets, 2013; Walter, 2006), as the use of such signals is a characteristic and critical feature of all mammal and most bird offspring (Newman, 2007). However, in animals and human newborns, this is a pure acoustical signal (i.e., human infants do not produce emotional tears in the first weeks of their lives), with only humans shedding emotional tears. Further, humans show tears throughout their lifespan, while most other species exhibit their comparable distress vocalizations mainly as young offspring.

DEVELOPMENTAL ASPECTS

Crying undergoes several important changes throughout the lifespan (Rottenberg & Vingerhoets, 2012; Zeifman, 2001). For example, crying tends to decrease in frequency from infancy until adolescence, and there is an increase in the significance of visual tears and a decrease in vocalizations (Provine, 2012). We also observe developmental changes in the antecedents of crying (Vingerhoets, 2013), as well as the development of gender differences (Jellesma & Vingerhoets, 2012).

Regarding the developmental changes in visual tears and vocalizations, we must look to humans' unique extended childhood, which allows the immature brain to freely and optimally develop. However, this extended childhood also makes human children vulnerable, requiring care, love, and protection from others well into the lifespan (Kipp, 1991/2008). Acoustical crying (i.e., vocalizations), as an attachment behavior, satisfies these needs by maintaining the proximity of the parent (i.e., crying as the "acoustical umbilical cord": Ostwald, 1972) and by soliciting care and assistance (Bowlby, 1980). This attachment function of crying is thought to continue throughout the lifespan, but shifts from vocalizations to tearful crying. A recent finding that adult tears have a stronger impact on observers than those of infants (Zeifman & Brown, 2011) supports the notion that tears replace the acoustical crying of infants over time. A significant advantage of tears over vocalizations comes from their capability to be targeted to individuals in close interactions, without notifying unwanted listeners of one's weakness or helplessness. Thus, as soon as an infant has acquired the motoric skills to move independently, we begin to see increases in visual tears.

The developmental changes in the reasons why humans cry appear to be, at least partially, related to other ongoing normal developmental processes (Zeifman, 2001). For example, the phenomenon of stranger anxiety—whereby infants cry when exposed to strangers—peaks toward the end of the first year. As children age, with the development of feelings of guilt, remorse, empathy, and the ability to take another's perspective ("theory of mind"), children may also cry, not only due to egocentric reasons, but because they can imagine and sympathize with the suffering of others. From infancy until adolescence, physical pain and discomfort are very important triggers of tears, but for adults and the elderly, these no longer play a significant role. On the other hand, feelings of loss and powerlessness remain important for crying at all ages. In addition, older adults show a greater tendency to cry due to positive situations, particularly in conjunction with experiences that give their lives depth and meaning, such as the intensification of relationships, altruism, and self-sacrifice (Cova & Deonna, 2013; Denckla, Fiori, & Vingerhoets, 2014; Rottenberg & Vingerhoets, 2012; Vingerhoets, 2013). The development of crying over the lifespan can thus be understood as starting from solely egocentric reasons (e.g., physical discomfort) and expanding over time to include societal (e.g., sentimental or moral) reasons. Along these lines, Vingerhoets (2013) outlines five types of emotional tears based on their antecedents, beginning from those more prominent in early development: (1) physical pain tears; (2) (egocentric) attachment-related pain tears; (3) empathic, compassionate pain tears; (4) societal pain tears; and (5) sentimental or morally based tears.

ANTECEDENTS AND CONTEXT OF ADULT EMOTIONAL CRYING

When adults are asked what triggered their most recent crying episode, the situations they typically report include conflicts, minor personal failures, criticism, rejection, sad music, and sentimental movies (Vingerhoets, 2013). Although one might think that major emotional events, such as the death of a loved one, divorce, physical pain, weddings, or the birth of a child, would be reported as the primary triggers for crying, these strongest elicitors of tears are quite rare in most humans' lives. Thus, we cry most often for more mundane and idiosyncratic reasons, which are largely dependent on personal and situational context, and which do not appear to have a strong, universal tear-eliciting capacity. Indeed, exposure to an emotional event by itself often is not sufficient to elicit tears—the person likely needs to be in a particular mental and/or physical state and situational context for tears to come.

In addition to situational antecedents, there are a wide variety of emotional states that may mediate the relationship between situational antecedents and tears (Vingerhoets, Van Geleuken, Van Tilburg, & Van Heck, 1997). Feeling powerless/helpless is the most common emotional trigger, especially when combined with emotions such as sadness, anger, fear, frustration, or disappointment. In the case of positive emotions, tears are particularly associated with feeling overwhelmed with joy, elation, or gratitude. While it is impossible to create universal lists of crying-eliciting situations, there can be little doubt that helplessness and hopelessness have a strong, universal power to elicit tears, particularly when such emotional states are associated with attachment-related issues such as bereavement, romantic break-ups, or moves (Denckla et al., 2014; Vingerhoets, 2013).

Although crying has many common underlying themes, there are still a number of individual differences in crying behavior that have been observed in adults. One of the most notable of these is the significant gender difference in crying behavior. Recent data show that adult women cry on average two to five times a month, and men about once every two months, although there is considerable interindividual and intercultural variation (Rottenberg, Bylsma, Wolvin, & Vingerhoets, 2008; Van Hemert, Vijver, & Vingerhoets, 2011; Vingerhoets, 2013; Vingerhoets & Scheirs, 2000). Regarding antecedents, women tend to cry more in conflict situations ("powerless anger"), whereas men cry relatively more often due to positive reasons (Vingerhoets, 2013). In the case of more dramatic situations (bereavement, romantic break-up, homesickness), the gender differences in crying are limited.

Individual differences in crying also depend on other variables, including personality factors, attachment style, mental health, culture, socialization, whether or not one is in a romantic relationship, and previous exposure to traumatic events. For example, individuals with high levels of neuroticism, extraversion, and empathy tend to cry more (Rottenberg, Bylsma, Wolvin, & Vingerhoets, 2008; Vingerhoets, 2013; Vingerhoets, Boelhouwer, Van Tilburg, & Van Heck, 2001), whereas dismissively attached persons cry relatively less (Laan, Van Assen, & Vingerhoets, 2012).

Bekker and Vingerhoets (2001; see also Vingerhoets, 2013) developed a model to illustrate that each of the following four factors (including combinations of factors) likely contribute to individual and group differences in crying. First, individuals or groups may have different degrees of exposure to emotional situations (e.g., women or individuals in romantic relationships may have more exposure to emotional situations, both in leisure time (e.g., a gender-specific selection of emotional movies or literature, arguments with one's romantic partner) and work settings (e.g., more women work in health care and men in technical and other less social professions)). Second, individuals or groups may differ in the way they appraise potentially emotional situations. Third, individuals likely have different crying thresholds, which may be related to physical and psychological factors, including health status, hormonal changes, and sleep deprivation. Finally, the fourth factor is the (learned) capacity to control one's tears and, relatedly, the social acceptance of tears.

FUNCTIONS OF HUMAN EMOTIONAL CRYING

There are a number of theories about the functions of human emotional tears. These theories generally fit into two broad categories: (1) intraindividual: those focusing on the effects of crying on the crier him- or herself, and (2) interindividual: those addressing the effects of crying on others.

Intraindividual Effects

Theories focusing on the *intraindividual* effects of crying primarily originate from the psychodynamic tradition and are strongly connected to the concept of catharsis (e.g., Breuer & Freud, 1895/1955; Bylsma, Vingerhoets, & Rottenberg, 2008; Koestler, 1964; Sadoff, 1966). According to these views, the production of tears is considered to be a sort of safety valve, serving to release superfluous emotional energy. Similarly, other theorists view crying as a method of releasing or discharging tension that has been built up by emotions inhibited from expression or with which an individual cannot otherwise properly cope (Bindra, 1972; Miceli & Castelfranchi, 2003). Tears, thus, may reflect feelings that cannot be expressed or consummated in other behaviors. Such theories of crying postulate that if this built-up tension is not released via tears, it may have a negative impact on bodily functioning and cause psychosomatic dysfunction. Thus, crying is considered cathartic and believed to result in mood improvement following crying, which promotes one's health, whereas the inhibition of emotional tears is seen as detrimental to physical functioning. There is some limited evidence that suppressing tears may have negative mental and physical effects (Bylsma et al., 2008; Vingerhoets & Bylsma, 2007a).

Irrespective of the real intraindividual effects of crying, beliefs about the cathartic benefits of crying may influence how individuals use their crying for mood management. For example, Simons, Bruder, van der Lowe, and Parkinson (2013) found that, when participants were asked about the reasons why they sometimes continue crying in sad or upsetting situations, they reported primarily doing so for the anticipated personal benefit or relief (rather than to influence the behavior of others). Also, in a recent study by Hanser, Ter Bogt, Van Tol, Mark, and Vingerhoets (2016), crying was reported to be the second (next to listening to specific music) most frequent behavior displayed when one is in need of self-comfort.

Moreover, Cornelius (1986) examined popular magazine articles spanning 140 years regarding the health effects of crying and found that 94% of the identified articles qualified crying as beneficial for one's well-being, even warning readers that suppressing tears could be deleterious to the body and mind. However, the empirical literature reveals a rather complex pattern of findings concerning the effects of crying on mood and well-being (Rottenberg, Bylsma, & Vingerhoets, 2008), with results heavily dependent upon the research methodology employed (Bylsma et al., 2008; Gračanin, Bylsma, & Vingerhoets, 2014; Rottenberg, Bylsma, & Vingerhoets, 2008). For example, an international study on adult crying (ISAC), containing survey data from over 5,000 men and women from 37 countries, found a strong consensus among respondents that crying helps them to feel better (>70%). However, when asked specifically about their most recent crying episode, only about half of these very same respondents reported experiencing a positive mood change after crying (Bylsma et al., 2008; Vingerhoets, 2013). In addition, in a study in which women completed daily mood diaries that included their crying episodes from that day, the reports of mood benefits after crying were just around 30% (Bylsma, Croon, Vingerhoets, & Rottenberg, 2011). And in quasi-experimental studies in which volunteers were exposed to sad movies, the participants who cried always felt worse immediately after the film (Cornelius, 1997).

It seems plausible that whether or not someone experiences benefits from crying also depends on *when* the individual is asked. In a quasi-experimental study, Gračanin, Vingerhoets, Kardum, Zupčić, Šantek, and Šimić (2015) evaluated mood immediately after participants watched a sad film, as well as over the course of 90 minutes following the film. Their findings confirmed those of previous laboratory studies demonstrating that crying results in poorer reported mood immediately following a sad movie. However, most critical was their observation that the decrease in mood was subsequently followed by a recovery after 20 and 90 minutes, with criers' self-reported mood after 90 minutes being even better than their baseline mood measured prior to the movie (and thus, importantly, prior to crying). The non-criers did not exhibit this pattern. These findings appear to reconcile the seemingly contradictory observations based on laboratory and retrospective studies. In laboratory studies using films to elicit tears, the participants provided mood ratings immediately after the crying episode, allowing no time for potential slower processes that result in mood benefits to take place. These new findings suggest that the benefits of crying may require more time to develop or, alternatively, that people develop more biases in how they think about crying as the time goes by.

Rottenberg, Bylsma, and Vingerhoets (2008), after examining the question of the influence of crying on mood, eventually concluded that the question "Is crying beneficial?" should be reformulated as follows: "For whom, and in what conditions, does crying benefit the crying individual?" Contributing factors that may influence whether or not crying is beneficial include the crier's personality and psychological state (e.g., individuals who are depressed rarely report mood improvement), characteristics of the eliciting event (when events are not in the crier's control, mood tends not to improve), and how others react to the crying (when criers receive comfort they tend to report mood improvement, whereas disapproval and other negative reactions are not associated with mood improvement; Rottenberg, Bylsma, & Vingerhoets, 2008).

Interpersonal Functions and Effects of Human Emotional Crying

Earlier we mentioned Bowlby's (1980) attachment theory regarding the functions of (infant) crying. Nelson (2005) expanded this view to assert that the help-soliciting function of crying is not only relevant for infants but is maintained throughout the lifespan into adulthood. Thus, crying has evolved—in children and adults—to be directed to attachment figures in order to elicit their attention and support. Hasson (2009) studied the functions of adult tears from an evolutionary perspective and hypothesized that tears serve an important interpersonal function, including promoting social bonding and inhibiting aggression in others. Anthropological literature on ritual weeping—similar to ritual praying or singing—suggests that such crying facilitates social bonding and stimulates feelings of mutual connectedness, especially in times of suffering (famine, natural disasters, war; Dissayanake, 2008; Vingerhoets, 2013).

There have been several research methods used in attempting to study the interpersonal effects of crying. A number of recent laboratory studies have used photographs of (crying) individuals and the same pictures with tears digitally removed or added (Balsters, Krahmer, Swerts, & Vingerhoets, 2013; Cornelius & Lubliner, 2003; Cornelius, Nussbaum, Warner, & Moeller, 2000; Provine, Krosnowski, & Brocato, 2009; Vingerhoets et al., 2016; Zeifman & Brown, 2011). These studies typically conclude that tearless (but otherwise crying) faces produce confusion about the emotional state of the individual, whereas visible tears have a positive effect on attributed kindness, feelings of empathy and connectedness, and the self-reported willingness to provide support. A limited number of laboratory studies (see Cornelius, 2001, for a review) have explored the social effects of tears by having confederates pretend to cry. These studies have generally found that crying confederates are evaluated less positively (i.e., more depressed and emotional) but also tend to elicit more sympathy than non-crying confederates. Overall, the research on how observers respond to a crying adult has found evidence from questionnaires, vignette studies, workplace studies, and laboratory studies that crying generally elicits supportive reactions from others, especially in the case of female criers (Bylsma et al., 2008; Hendriks, Croon, & Vingerhoets, 2008; Vingerhoets, Van de Ven, & Van der Velden, 2016).

Some situational and contextual factors have been found to be important in predicting the reactions of others to crying individuals. In the ISAC study mentioned earlier, participants were asked how others had responded to their last crying episode (Bylsma et al., 2008; Vingerhoets, 2013). Results showed that the nature of the relationship with the crying individual was a major determinant of the reactions, with close individuals being more likely to provide comfort and support, especially physically. Plas and Hoover Dempsey (1988) found, through interviews, that crying in an intimate setting is generally accepted, but in the work setting it may be more likely to trigger negative reactions in colleagues.

Vingerhoets (2013) outlined a model that summarizes the putative factors that appear to determine reactions to observed crying: (1) the situation and its perceived appropriateness as an elicitor of crying; (2) the characteristics of the crying person: age, gender, personality, status, and specific role (e.g., caregiver, politician, health professional); (3) the characteristics of the observer: age, gender, personality, professional status; (4) the characteristics of the relationship between the observer and the crying person: whether it concerns a communal relationship (e.g., friendship, intimate relationship), exchange (e.g., business relationship), or professional help provision (e.g., physician, psychotherapist); and (5) the specific characteristics of the crying (e.g., protest crying, sad crying, or mere tearfulness).

CRYING AND HEALTH

Crying has been associated with several aspects of mental and physical health (Vingerhoets & Bylsma, 2007a, 2007b). More specifically, changes in crying may be a symptom, a sign, or a consequence of certain diseases and their treatment.

Neurological disorders (e.g., stroke, multiple sclerosis) and endocrine diseases (e.g., thyroid disorders) are well known for their possible effects on an individual's crying behavior (Vingerhoets, 2013). Regarding mental health, several psychiatric disorders, including mood disorders, anxiety disorders, and schizophrenia, have been associated with more frequent crying. Depression is also associated with changes in crying, although the nature of that relationship is not totally clear. While some studies demonstrate increased crying in depressed samples (e.g., Frey, Hoffman-Ahern, Johnson, Lykken, & Tuason, 1983; Hastrup, Baker, Kraemer, & Bornsetin, 1986; Rottenberg, Cevaal, & Vingerhoets, 2008), others find no relationship between depression levels and crying (Rottenberg, Gross, Willhelm, Najmi, & Gotlib, 2002). Still others suggest a non-linear relationship between depression and crying, with severe levels of depression associated with less frequent crying or even the loss of the ability to cry, but mild or moderate levels of depression associated with increased crying, as reflected in the scoring of the Beck Depression Inventory crying item (Vingerhoets, Rottenberg, Cevaal, & Nelson, 2007). Keller and Nesse (2005) propose a link between the etiology of depression and crying behavior. According to this view, when depression occurs due to significant loss, crying is a major symptom, but when depression results from a high workload or chronic stress, other symptoms (e.g., fatigue) may prevail. In addition, it has been suggested that depressed individuals may experience fewer mood benefits from crying (Rottenberg, Bylsma, & Vingerhoets, 2008), indicating the possible impairment of regulatory functions of crying.

CRYING IN THE THERAPY CONTEXT

Similar to the general public, psychotherapists and counselors from various traditions and backgrounds have considered crying by the client during therapy to be constructive, rather than destructive (Blume-Marcovici, Stolberg, & Khademi, 2013; 't Lam, 2011), as well as a positive attachment experience for clients in which they have the chance to receive attuned caregiving in response to their tears (Nelson, 2005). In one study, over 70% of clinicians reported that they actively encourage their clients to cry (Trezza, Hastrup, & Kim, 1988).

Some research has investigated the impact of client crying depending on particular client traits. Alexander (2003) found that therapists in clinical settings may perceive the crying of clients with borderline or narcissistic personality disorders as manipulative or annoying, even potentially inducing such strongly negative feelings in therapists that the development of empathy and rapport is adversely affected. Robinson, Hill, and Kivlighan (2015) found that both clients' and therapists' attachment styles influence the frequency and type of crying in therapy, and the authors suggest that crying is a specific form of communication to which the therapist should be particularly attuned. They also point out that therapists should not assume crying to be inherently positive or negative.

It may be helpful to consider the following research findings in the context of clients' tears in therapy: (1) helplessness is a primary emotion experienced when individuals cry (Denckla et al., 2014); (2) individuals prefer to cry in the presence of "attachment figures" such as one's mother or romantic partner (Fox, 2004); and (3) individuals appear to encourage their own crying in order to elicit support from others and consequently relieve their own distress (Simons et al., 2013). Considering these factors, a client's act of crying might be (prototypically) interpreted as sending messages of: (1) being in need of help; (2) feeling close to the therapist; and (3) implicit expectancy of a supportive, empathic reaction and consequent relief. When it comes to the empathic response, therapists may sometimes also cry in the therapy context. Research on this specific phenomenon is presented in Chapter 2 of this volume, but it is worth noting here that a study of therapist crying in daily life (outside of therapy) found therapists to have a higher crying tendency than the general public, with the same pattern of gender differences (i.e., female therapists cried more frequently than male therapists; 't Lam & Vingerhoets, 2016). There are a number of reasons therapists may cry more than individuals in the general public, such as: (1) therapists may be higher on personality variables, such as empathy, that increase their tendency to cry; (2) therapists may be more comfortable with their own tears; (3) therapists may have increased awareness of their tendency to cry; and (4) therapists may have more exposure to situations that elicit crying given the nature of their work.

CONCLUSION

Tearful crying appears to facilitate social bonding, elicit sympathy, promote cooperative and helpful behavior, and inhibit aggression (Hasson, 2009; Vingerhoets, 2013; Walter 2006). Tears are a sign to others that we are in need of help and support; therefore, they represent an important mechanism that is at the basis of our social functioning. Indeed, emotional tears, as a form of attachment behavior, may have contributed to our development into an ultrasocial species. Tears often accompany our experience of our most important life events, both positive and negative. From this perspective, the role of adult tears may be to alert the crier to the fact that the situation to which he or she is exposed is an important one, not only for the crier him- or herself, but for society at large. In this way, emotional crying, as a ubiquitous, poignant, mysterious, and uniquely human behavior, is something to which we can all relate.

NOTE

1. For a complete literature review on several of these topics, see our recent overview of human emotional crying: Vingerhoets, A. J. J. M, & Bylsma, L. M. (2015). The riddle of human emotional crying: A challenge for emotion researchers, *Emotion Review*, 1–11.

REFERENCES

Alexander, T. (2003). Narcissism and the experience of crying. *British Journal of Psychotherapy, 20*, 27–37.

Balsters, M., Krahmer, E., Swerts, M., & Vingerhoets, A. J. J. M. (2013). Emotional tears facilitate the recognition of sadness and the perceived need for social support. *Evolutionary Psychology, 11*, 148–158.

Bekker, M. H. J., & Vingerhoets, A. J. J. M. (2001). Male and female tears: Swallowing versus shedding? The relationship between crying, biological sex and gender. In A. J. J. M. Vingerhoets & R. R. Cornelius (Eds.), *Adult crying: A biopsychosocial approach* (pp. 91–114). Hove, UK: Brunner-Routledge.

Bindra, D. (1972). Weeping: A problem of many facets. *Bulletin of the British Psychological Society, 25,* 281–285.

Blume-Marcovici, A. C., Stolberg, R. A., & Khademi, M. (2013). Do therapists cry in therapy? The role of experience and other factors in therapists' tears. *Psychotherapy, 50,* 224–234.

Bowlby, J. (1980). *Loss: Sadness and depression.* New York, NY: Basic Books.

Breuer, J., & Freud, S. (1895/1955). *Studies on hysteria* (trans. J. Strachey). London: Hogarth Press (1955 edition).

Bylsma, L. M., Croon, M. A., Vingerhoets, A. J. J. M., & Rottenberg, J. (2011). When and for whom does crying improve mood? A daily diary study of 1004 crying episodes. *Journal of Research in Personality, 45,* 385–392.

Bylsma, L. M., Vingerhoets, A. J. J. M., & Rottenberg, J. (2008). When is crying cathartic? An international study. *Journal of Social and Clinical Psychology, 27,* 1165–1187.

Cornelius, R. R. (1986). *Prescience in the pre-scientific study of weeping? A history of weeping in the popular press from the mid-1800s to the present.* Paper presented at the 75th Annual Meeting of the Eastern Psychological Association, New York.

Cornelius, R. R. (1997). Toward a new understanding of weeping and catharsis? In A. J. J. M. Vingerhoets, F. J. Van Bussel, & A. J. W. Boelhouwer (Eds.), *The (non)expression of emotions in health and disease* (pp. 303–321). Tilburg: Tilburg University Press.

Cornelius, R. R. (2001). Crying and catharsis. In A. J. J. M. Vingerhoets & R. R. Cornelius (Eds.), *Adult crying: A biopsychosocial approach* (pp. 199–212). Hove, UK: Brunner-Routledge.

Cornelius, R. R., & Lubliner, E. (2003, October). *The what and why of others' responses to our tears: Adult crying as an attachment behavior.* Paper presented at the third international conference on the (Non)Expression of Emotions in Health and Disease, Tilburg, the Netherlands.

Cornelius, R. R., Nussbaum, R., Warner, L., & Moeller, C. (2000, August). *"An action full of meaning and of real service": The social and emotional messages of crying.* Paper presented at the 11th conference of the International Society for Research on Emotions, Quebec City, Canada.

Cova, F., & Deonna, J. A. (2013). Being moved. *Philosophical Studies, 169,* 447–466.

Darwin, C. (1872). *The expression of the emotions in man and animals.* New York, NY: Oxford University Press (1998 edition, with an introduction, afterword and commentaries by P. Ekman).

Denckla, C. A., Fiori, K. L., & Vingerhoets, A. J. J. M. (2014). Development of the crying proneness scale: Associations among crying proneness, empathy, attachment, and age. *Journal of Personality Assessment, 96,* 619–631.

Dissayanake, E. (2008). If music is the food of love, what about survival and reproductive success? *Musicae Scientiae, Special Issue 1*, 169–195.

Fox, K. (2004). *The Kleenex © for Men crying game report: A study of men and crying.* Oxford, UK: Social Issues Research Center.

Frey, W. H., Hoffman-Ahern, C., Johnson, R. A., Lykken, D. T., & Tuason, V. B. (1983). Crying behavior in the human adult. *Integrative Psychiatry, 1*(3), 94–98.

Gračanin, A., Bylsma, L., & Vingerhoets, A. J. J. M. (2014). Is crying a self-soothing behaviour? *Frontiers in Psychology, 5*, 502.

Gračanin, A., Vingerhoets, A. J. J. M., Kardum, I., Zupčić, M., Šantek, M., & Šimić, M. (2015). Why crying does and sometimes does not seem to alleviate mood: A quasi-experimental study. *Motivation and Emotion, 39*, 953–960.

Hanser, W. E., Ter Bogt, T. F. M., Van Tol, A. J. M., Mark, R. E., & Vingerhoets, A. J. J. M. (2016). Consolation through music: A survey study. *Musicae Scientiae*, 1–16.

Hasson, O. (2009). Emotional tears as biological signals. *Evolutionary Psychology, 7*, 363–370.

Hastrup, J. L., Baker, J. G., Kraemer, D. L., & Bornstein, R. F. (1986). Crying and depression among older adults. *The Gerontologist, 26*(1), 91.

Hendriks, M. C. P., Croon, M. A., & Vingerhoets, A. J. J. M. (2008). Social reactions to adult crying: The help-soliciting function of tears. *Journal of Social Psychology, 148*, 22–41.

Jellesma, F. C., & Vingerhoets, A. J. J. M. (2012). Crying in middle childhood: A report on gender differences. *Sex Roles, 6–7*, 412–421.

Keller, M. C., & Nesse, R. M. (2005). Is low mood an adaptation? Evidence for subtypes with symptoms that match precipitants. *Journal of Affective Disorders, 86*, 27–35.

Kipp, F. (1991; 2008). *Die Evolution des Menschen im Hinblick auf seine lange Jugendzeit.* Translated by J.M. Barnes: Childhood and human evolution. Hillsdale, NJ: Adonis Press.

Koestler, A. (1964). *The act of creation.* London, UK: Hutchinson.

Laan, A., Van Assen, M. A. L., & Vingerhoets, A. J. J. M. (2012). Individual differences in adult crying: The role of attachment styles. *Social Behavior and Personality, 40*, 453–471.

Miceli, M., & Castelfranchi, C. (2003). Crying: Discussing its basic reasons and uses. *New Ideas in Psychology, 21*, 247–273.

Murube, J. (2009). Hypotheses on the development of psychoemotional tearing. *The Ocular Surface, 7*, 171–175.

Nelson, J. K. (2005). *Seeing through tears: Crying and attachment.* New York, NY: Routledge.

Newman, J. D. (2007). Neural circuits underlying crying and cry responding in mammals. *Behavioural Brain Research, 182*(2), 155–165.

Ostwald, P. (1972). The sounds of infancy. *Developmental Medicine and Child Neurology, 14*, 350–361.

Patel, V. (1993). Crying behavior and psychiatric disorder in adults: A review. *Comprehensive Psychiatry, 34*, 206–211.

Plas, J. M., & Hoover Dempsey, K. V. (1988). *Working up a storm: Anger, anxiety, joy, and tears on the job.* New York, NY: W.W. Norton.

Provine, R. R. (2012). *Curious behavior: Yawning, laughing, hiccupping, and beyond.* Cambridge, MA: The Belknap Press.

Provine, R. R., Krosnowski, K. A., & Brocato, N. W. (2009). Tearing: Breakthrough in human emotional signaling. *Evolutionary Psychology, 7*, 52–56.

Robinson, N., Hill, C. E., & Kivlighan, D. M. (2015). Crying as communication in psychotherapy: The influence of client and therapist attachment dimensions and client attachment to therapist on amount and type of crying. *Journal of Counseling Psychology, 62*, 379–392.

Rottenberg, J., Bylsma, L. M., & Vingerhoets, A. J. J. M. (2008). Is crying beneficial? *Current Directions in Psychological Science, 17*, 400–404.

Rottenberg, J., Bylsma, L. M., Wolvin, V., & Vingerhoets, A. J. J. M. (2008). Tears of sorrow, tears of joy: An individual differences approach to crying in Dutch females. *Personality and Individual Differences, 45*, 367–372.

Rottenberg, J., Cevaal, A., & Vingerhoets, A. J. J. M. (2008). Do mood disorders alter crying? A pilot investigation. *Depression and Anxiety, 25*, 9–15.

Rottenberg, J., Gross, J. J., Wilhelm, F. H., Najmi, S., & Gotlib, I. H. (2002). Crying threshold and intensity in major depressive disorder. *Journal of Abnormal Psychology, 111*, 302–312.

Rottenberg, J., & Vingerhoets, A. J. J. M. (2012). Crying: Call for a developmental lifespan approach. *Personality and Social Psychology Compass, 6*, 217–227.

Sadoff, R. L. (1966). On the nature of crying and weeping. *Psychiatric Quarterly, 40*, 490–503.

Simons, G., Bruder, M., van der Lowe, I., & Parkinson, B. (2013). Why try (not) to cry: Intra- and inter-personal motives for crying regulation. *Frontiers in Psychology, 3*, 1–9.

't Lam, C. (2011). *Attitudes ten aanzien van en ervaringen met huilen tijdens therapie. Een onderzoek onder hulpverleners. {Attitudes towards and experiences with crying during therapy. A study among mental health professionals.}* Unpublished Master's thesis. Tilburg, the Netherlands: Clinical Psychology Section, Tilburg School of Social and Behavioral Sciences.

't Lam, C., & Vingerhoets, A. J. J. M. (2016). De tranen van de therapeut. [The tears of the therapist.] *De Psycholoog, 7*, 10–20.

Trezza, G. R., Hastrup, J. L., & Kim, S. E. (1988). *Clinicians' attitudes and beliefs about crying behavior*. Paper presented at the Eastern Psychological Association Annual Meeting, Buffalo, NY.

Trimble, M. (2012). *Why humans like to cry: Tragedy, evolution, and the brain*. Oxford, UK: Oxford University Press.

Van Hemert, D., Van de Vijver, F., & Vingerhoets, A. J. J. M. (2011). Culture and crying: Prevalences and gender differences. *Cross-Cultural Research, 45*, 399–431.

Vingerhoets, A. J. J. M. (2013). *Why only humans weep: Unraveling the mysteries of tears*. Oxford, UK: Oxford University Press.

Vingerhoets, A. J. J. M., Boelhouwer, A. J. W., van Tilburg, M. A. L., & van Heck, G. L. (2001). The situational and emotional context of adult crying. In A. J. J. M. Vingerhoets, & R. R. Cornelius (Eds.), *Adult crying: A biopsychosocial approach* (pp. 71–90). Hove, UK: Brunner-Routledge.

Vingerhoets, A. J. J. M., & Bylsma, L. M. (2007a). Crying as a multifaceted health psychology conceptualisation: Crying as coping, risk factor, and symptom. *The European Health Psychologist, 9*, 68–74.

Vingerhoets, A. J. J. M., & Bylsma, L. M. (2007b). Crying and health: Popular and scientific conceptions. *Psihologijske Teme, 16*.

Vingerhoets, A. J. J. M., & Bylsma, L. M. (2015). The riddle of human emotional crying: A challenge for emotion researchers. *Emotion Review*, 1–11.

Vingerhoets, A. J. J. M., van Geleuken, A. J. M. L., van Tilburg, M. A. L., & van Heck, G. L. (1997). The psychological context of crying episodes: Towards a model of adult crying. In A. J. J. M. Vingerhoets, F. van Bussel, & A. Boelhouwer (Eds.), *The (non)expression of emotions in health and disease* (pp. 323–336). Tilburg: Tilburg University Press.

Vingerhoets, A., Rottenberg, J., Cevaal, A., & Nelson, J. K. (2007). Is there a relationship between depression and crying? A review. *Acta Psychiatrica Scandinavica, 115*(5), 340–351.

Vingerhoets, A. J. J. M., & Scheirs, J. (2000). Sex differences in crying: Empirical findings and possible explanations. In A. H. Fischer (Ed.), *Gender and emotion: Social psychological perspectives* (pp. 143–165). Cambridge: Cambridge University Press.

Vingerhoets, A. J. J. M., Van de Ven, N., & Van der Velden, Y. (2016). The social impact of emotional tears. *Motivation and Emotion*. Advance online publication.

Walter, C. (2006). *Thumbs, toes, and tears: And other traits that make us human*. New York, NY: Walker.

Zeifman, D. M. (2001). Developmental aspects of crying: Infancy, childhood and beyond. In A. J. J. M. Vingerhoets & R. R. Cornelius (Eds.), *Adult crying: A biopsychosocial perspective* (pp. 37–53). Hove, UK: Brunner-Routledge.

Zeifman, D. M., & Brown, S. A. (2011). Age-related changes in the signal value of tears. *Evolutionary Psychology, 9*, 313–324.

CHAPTER 2

TRACKING OUR TEARS: RESEARCH ON THERAPIST CRYING IN THERAPY

Amy Blume-Marcovici, Ronald A. Stolberg, Mojgan Khademi, Anthony Mackie, and Catelijne 't Lam

Clients cry in psychotherapy. Indeed, their tears are a valued event in the therapy hour, with research showing that the vast majority of mental health professionals believe that client tears are important for the therapeutic process ('t Lam & Vingerhoets, 2016). As a testament to the valuation—even expectation—of client tears in therapy, one of the authors of this chapter recalls running—literally—to a pharmacy between client sessions when realizing the office tissue stash had been depleted. But do therapists—the ones with whom clients share their tears—ever themselves cry in therapy?

For some therapists, the intuitive answer is *of course*. They feel it would be unreasonable or callous to expect that tears would never come to their eyes when witnessing the suffering, or the profound healing, of another soul. For others, their immediate response is: *"There's no crying in therapy—for the therapist!"* For this group, the idea that therapists may indulge in their own emotional expressions in a session is a breach of professionalism and a sign that the therapist is not able to adequately focus on the needs of the client, even that the therapist him- or herself should go to therapy. It is likely that the majority of therapists fall somewhere in between. But how often does therapist crying in therapy really occur? What do therapists feel about their own tearfulness in sessions? And what do their clients feel about their therapist's tears? In this chapter, we will review the research that exists regarding therapists' crying in therapy in an attempt to illuminate the trends and diversity in therapists' and clients' beliefs about and perceptions of therapists' tears.

TEARS IN THERAPY: THE RESEARCH

Do Therapists Cry?

While only a handful of studies have directly investigated the frequency of therapists' tears in therapy, each one has concluded that the majority of therapists have experienced tearfulness at some point during a therapy session with a client. Pope, Tabachnick, and Keith-Spiegel (1987) found that, of the 456 psychologists who responded to their survey on ethical behaviors, just over half (57%) reported that they had cried in the presence of a client. Tritt, Kelly, and Waller (2015), in a study that investigated therapist crying from clients' perspectives, also found that 57% of 188 clients in their study reported that their therapist had cried during the course of treatment. Brownlie (2014) surveyed 439 Australian registered psychologists and found that 62% reported having cried in therapy. In a survey of 19 psychodynamic therapists, Nelson (2007) found that two-thirds had cried in a session. Seventy-two percent of the 684 U.S. psychologists and psychology trainees that Blume-Marcovici, Stolberg, and Khademi (2013) surveyed in their study on therapist crying reported having cried in therapy. And 't Lam and Vingerhoets (2016), in their study of 819 Dutch mental health professionals' experiences with tears, found that 87% had cried while conducting therapy. From these data, we can see that many therapists do at times tear up and cry during therapy sessions. In fact, most have experienced this phenomenon.

How Often Do Therapists Cry in Therapy?

Of those therapists who have cried in therapy, the frequency of tearfulness ranges from extremely rare to relatively common. Pope et al. (1987) found that, while only 0.07% of their survey respondents reported having cried "very often" in therapy (that's about 32 of the 456 psychologists in their study), 41.5% (or 189) reported they cried "rarely." Nelson (2007) observed that 10% of her psychodynamic therapist research participants described crying "frequently," which she defined as once or twice a month, while the majority who cried reported doing so "rarely." 't Lam and Vingerhoets (2016) investigated crying frequency in therapy based on levels of crying intensity and found that over one-third of respondents had tears in their eyes at least ten times in the last year, and 75% had teared up at least five times in the last year.

In looking at the frequency of therapist crying as a percentage of total therapy sessions, Blume-Marcovici et al. (2013) found that psychologists and psychology trainees experienced tearfulness in approximately 7% of therapy sessions. Compared to a study of client crying (Trezza, Hastrup, & Kim, 1988), which found, per therapists' report, that clients had "watery eyes" in 21% of therapy sessions, "some tears" in 15%, "many tears" in 9%, and "sobbing" in 3% of sessions, these data suggest that therapists tear up or cry in therapy almost one-third as often as their clients. A more recent study of client crying (Robinson, Hill, & Kivlighan, 2015) found client tears in approximately 14% of sessions, based on coding by independent raters. Compared to this figure, therapists experienced tearfulness about half as often as their clients. Of course, this is not taking intensity or longevity of tears into account and we can surmise that therapists' tears are less intense and more fleeting (i.e., tearfulness) than those of their clients'.

Above we have described research on the frequency of therapists' tears from the therapist's perspective. Another way of understanding the frequency with which therapists cry in therapy is from the client's recollection. Tritt et al. (2015) surveyed 188 clients who had completed a course of psychotherapy for an eating disorder and asked them to report the number of therapist crying episodes during the entire course of their completed treatment. Clients reported their therapists to have "looked or sounded close to tears" an average of 4.2 times across the course of therapy and that the therapist "cried openly but was able to carry on" an average of 1.64 times ($SD = 5.1$). While clients did report that their therapist sometimes cried openly and either had to pause the session or end the session as a result of crying, this was very rare ($M = 0.3$ and $M = 0.46$, respectively). Unfortunately, the authors did not collect data regarding the total number of therapist sessions in each treatment and therefore it is difficult to draw conclusions about frequency more specific than number of therapist crying episodes per course of treatment.

In What Therapeutic Context Do Therapists Cry in Therapy?

Type of Treatment

Based on client-reported rates of therapist crying during a completed course of treatment, Tritt et al. (2015) found no significant differences in crying between therapists who stated that they were delivering manual-based therapies versus non-manual-based approaches, though the authors note a trend in which those delivering non-manual-based psychotherapy may have cried more. In a study of 411 therapists' most recent experiences of crying in therapy, Blume-Marcovici, Stolberg, and Khademi (2015) found that the majority of crying episodes occurred in working with individual clients. While fewer crying episodes were reported in working with groups, couples, and families, the authors note that cases were reported in each of these settings. Thus it seems that therapist crying occurs in a range of treatments, from manual-based to less structured and from individual to group. However, therapist crying may be more likely to occur in non-manual-based, individual treatments.

Stage of Therapy

In a survey of therapists, Nelson's (2007) respondents believed that a therapist's tears early in treatment would be more detrimental than tears later in treatment, once the therapeutic attachment had been established and tears could be processed with more attunement to the client's specific needs. Conversely, Nelson's participants noted that tears early in treatment may lead to the client feeling "confused about [the] therapist's ability and capacities to manage [the client's] strong affects, which . . . [early in treatment can be] quite scary" (pp. 9–10). Mackie (2009) conducted a qualitative study in which he interviewed seven therapists (five psychologists and two counseling practitioners) about their experience of crying in a therapy session and found that, indeed, an existing close bond seemed to be an important prerequisite to therapists' tears emerging. In all but one instance, the therapists reported that their tears emerged in the presence of long-term clients with whom they had a strong emotional investment: these clients were "special" in some way to the therapists. Blume-Marcovici et al. (2015) similarly found that therapists were most likely to experience tearfulness in therapy "mid-treatment" or "late in treatment" and least likely to experience crying during an intake session, though the authors noted that this did occur. In addition, Nelson's research (2007) suggests that crying at terminations is more commonplace than at other stages of treatment and may help to account for the increased crying late in treatment that Blume-Marcovici et al. (2015) observed.

What Do Therapists Feel When They Cry?

In their study of therapists' most recent experiences of tearfulness in therapy, Blume-Marcovici et al. (2015) presented therapists with a list of 20 emotions and asked them to identify which they felt during their most recent crying episode (they could check more than one emotion). The most common emotions reported were: sadness (75%), feeling "touched" (63%), warmth (33%), loss (27%), powerlessness (15%), gratitude (15%), and joy (12%). The authors noted that, of the top seven most common emotional experiences, four were "positive," and three were "negative." The authors suggest that the emotions therapists feel when they cry may be more positive—or at least heterogeneous—in nature than one might initially assume. Indeed, Brownlie's (2014) study of 439 Australian registered psychologists found that participants were prone to crying specifically in response to positive emotional events and therapists' tears were often associated with positive relational emotions such as feelings of care, connection, or empathy. Similarly, in his qualitative study of therapists' experiences of crying in therapy, Mackie (2009) found that, while therapists reported a wide spectrum of emotional experiences alongside their tears—from sadness and anger to pride and joy—an overarching theme was that therapists described experiencing powerful feelings of companionship and affection for their client in these moments. These were also often accompanied by an inclination to physically approach or touch the client, which Mackie interpreted as evidence of attachment processes occurring in these moments.

Blume-Marcovici et al. (2015) also surveyed therapists regarding their feelings of comfort and/or regret when they cried in therapy. They found that, in most cases (59%), therapists felt comfortable with their tears. However, almost one-third (31%) of their respondents expressed discomfort with crying in therapy (the remainder remained neutral). Respondents also tended not to express regret or remorse at having cried, with only 9% wishing they had not cried and 4% believing their tears to have been a therapeutic mistake. The researchers described a correlation between regretting tears in therapy and reporting that one's tears were due to the therapist's own personal situation, as opposed to related to the client's situation. While most of the time, clinicians indicated that their tears were directly related to their attunement to their client's situation, in 16% of cases in Blume-Marcovici et al.'s (2015) study therapists reported that their crying was related to their own personal situation, and these latter therapists were more likely to report wishing they had not cried or feeling that their tears had been a mistake. Brownlie (2014) investigated this issue as well, examining whether therapist crying is a self-oriented emotional response (i.e., in reaction to personal experience and distress) or an other-oriented emotional response (i.e., related to witnessing another person's emotions). She found that therapists' tears were most commonly other-oriented. In other words, therapists in her study tended to experience their own tears as occurring in response to their connection to their client.

It appears that clients agree and most often interpret their therapist's tears as being related to the therapist empathizing with their (the client's) experience, i.e., as other-oriented (Tritt et al., 2015). However, if the therapist is perceived by the client to have a "negative demeanor," that is, the therapist is perceived by the client to be, in general, more anxious, bored, or angry during the therapy, clients tend to believe that their therapist's tears are related to something wrong in the therapist's own life (Tritt et al., 2015).

Which Therapists Cry in Therapy?

Theoretical Orientation

Clinicians who identify as specialists in cognitive-behavioral therapy (CBT) tend to report tearfulness in therapy significantly less than clinicians of any other theoretical orientation (Blume-Marcovici et al., 2013; Brownlie, 2014) and report a more negative attitude toward therapist crying ('t Lam & Vingerhoets, 2016). On the other hand, having a psychodynamic approach to therapy is associated with significantly higher rates of tears in therapy, with psychoanalysts ranking higher than any other therapeutic orientation (Blume-Marcovici et al., 2013). We may note that psychoanalysts sometimes use the couch, with their client in a recumbent position, which would conceal the analysts' tears and perhaps allow them to come more freely or frequently. While cognitive-behavioral clinicians tend to rate themselves as having lower rates of crying than other theoretical orientations, the same does not necessarily hold true for client ratings. Indeed, the most common type of therapy in which clients reported their therapist crying was CBT (Tritt et al., 2015). However, it is possible that there was simply a higher number of CBT therapists in the targeted sample and that, therefore, the data do not imply more frequent crying amongst CBT clinicians per se. Still, it is important to note that, while CBT therapists rate themselves as having the lowest crying rates, therapist crying does occur in all treatment settings.

Clinical Experience

The longer therapists have practiced therapy, the more frequently they report being tearful in therapy sessions (Blume-Marcovici et al., 2013; Brownlie, 2014) and the less conflicted they feel about their tears (Blume-Marcovici et al., 2013; 't Lam & Vingerhoets, 2016; Waldman, 1995). Indeed, 't Lam and Vingerhoets (2016) found that, over time, clinicians in their study came to have more positive attitudes toward therapist crying, came to see crying in therapy as a way to bond with clients and, overall, became more comfortable with crying as they became more comfortable and secure in their role as clinicians. Similarly, in a qualitative study on crying among psychodynamic therapists, Waldman (1995) found that her respondents' perception of therapists' affective displays in therapy changed over time, with clinicians feeling more comfortable during the later stages of their practice. Conversely, newer clinicians have more negative attitudes about crying and feel more regret about their tears (Blume-Marcovici et al., 2015; Waldman, 1995).

Why might this be? As respondents in 't Lam and Vingerhoets' (2016) and Waldman's (1995) research indicated, perhaps therapists become more comfortable using their clinical judgment in being less rigid and thus have fewer restrictions on their own affective displays. Blume-Marcovici et al. (2013) described an additional hypothesis which relates to both age of the therapist and the affective valence of the therapy sessions in which therapist crying occurs. In their study, they—not surprisingly—found that just as increased clinical experience correlated with increased crying, older clinicians reported higher rates of crying. In attempting to understand the relationship between clinical experience, age, and therapist crying in therapy, they noted that the older respondents in their study actually had *lower* crying rates in daily life (outside of therapy), a trend consistent with prior findings that individuals tend to cry less with age (Borquist, 1906; Williams & Morris, 1996). Thus, the direction of the correlation reversed in therapy, with increased age correlating with *higher* rates of crying in therapy but *lower* rates of crying outside of therapy.

However, the authors noted that on one subscale of the measure they used to assess crying in daily life (outside of therapy) there was a positive correlation between crying and age. This subscale measured proneness to cry due to positive situational antecedents, such as crying at weddings or the birth of a child, and crying due to feelings of rapture or that the world is just and good. So while the correlation between overall crying and age was significantly negative, the direction of the correlation reversed and was significantly positive when focusing only on crying due to positive situations. In other words, older individuals cried more in daily life owing to positive antecedents but less in daily life owing to negative antecedents. This is a trend that has been shown in other studies as well, in which older adults increasingly cry because of positive situations, particularly those experiences that give their lives a sense of meaning (Cova & Deonna, 2014; Denckla, Fiori, & Vingerhoets, 2014; Vingerhoets & Bylsma, 2016). Blume-Marcovici et al. (2013) speculated that this may explain the relationship between age, clinical experience, and therapist crying: the affective tone of scenarios in which clinicians cry in therapy may be more "positive" or "mixed" than the general scenarios in which individuals cry in their own day-to-day lives, thus contributing to increased rates of crying among older clinicians.

Sex

Males cry significantly less than females in day-to-day life (Bylsma, Vingerhoets, & Rottenberg, 2008; Vingerhoets & Bylsma, 2016). It is, thus, particularly striking that the studies on therapist crying in therapy have found no significant sex differences in rates of crying (Blume-Marcovici et al., 2013; Brownlie, 2014; 't Lam & Vingerhoets, 2016). Tritt et al. (2015) did find a significant difference in that female therapists were described by their clients as more likely than male therapists to "cry openly but carry on" in a session, while male therapists were more likely to have "cried and had to end the session" than female therapists. However, no significant differences were found between male and female therapists in frequency of "looking or sounding close to tears" or "crying openly and having to pause the session." Overall, research indicates that female and male therapists experience similar rates of tearfulness in therapy.

The explanations for this lack of sex difference in crying in therapy rates range from speculations that male therapists are less likely to adhere to strict gender role expectations regarding emotional expression when in therapy, perhaps even as a means of modeling appropriate affect, to findings that female therapists report higher rates of feeling the urge to cry and inhibiting their tears (i.e., females hold back tears in therapy more than males, while males are more likely to allow their tears to flow; Blume-Marcovici et al., 2013; 't Lam & Vingerhoets, 2016). In addition, 't Lam and Vingerhoets (2016) found that female therapists had a slightly but significantly more negative attitude toward therapists' crying than male therapists, which may account for why females are more likely to inhibit their tears and/or why males are more likely to let them flow.

The positive, or at least emotionally mixed, affective tone of many therapy sessions in which therapists cry may also help to explain this unexpected finding of equal crying rates amongst females and males (Blume-Marcovici et al., 2013). Previous researchers have found that when men cry in daily life, they tend to cry more because of positive reasons and emotional states (Bindra, 1972; Bylsma et al., 2008; Vingerhoets & Bylsma, 2016). Just as with age, it is possible that the relatively higher rates of crying among men in therapy, as opposed to daily life, can be explained by a more positive (or mixed) affective tone in therapy sessions in which tears in therapy occur.

While there do not appear to be significant sex differences in rates of crying in therapy, researchers have reported some differences regarding therapists' tears depending on the sex of the client. Blume-Marcovici et al. (2013) found that, overall, therapists reported crying more frequently with female than with male clients. However, when taking into account the sex of the therapist as well, they found that primarily female therapists were more likely to report crying with female clients, while male therapists were equally likely to report crying with male and female clients. In Waldman's (1995) qualitative study, respondents reported that their own tears were different with male and female clients. Some participants expressed concern that, because of women's societal role as caregivers, female clients may feel the need to take care of a crying therapist more than male clients. Others expressed that, because of the high value placed on the rarer commodity of male tears, sharing tears as a therapist with male clients may be an especially powerful experience. One male therapist, for instance, noted, "there is something special about sharing these moments with another man . . . it's really important for men to have models of emotional expression, and that men really respond to permission to feel" (Waldman, 1995, p. 87).

Personality

In their study of 684 psychologists and psychology trainees, Blume-Marcovici et al. (2013) found very small, somewhat equivocal, correlations between rates of crying in therapy and three of the Big Five personality traits: openness, agreeableness, and extraversion. Notably, when looking at their sample with regard to personality and crying in daily life, the personality trait of neuroticism (defined by the tendency to experience negative emotionality; John & Srivastava, 1999) correlated with increased crying in daily life but had no significant relationship with crying in therapy. The authors explained that the tendency to experience negative emotions (the definition of neuroticism as a personality trait) that correlated with crying in daily life was not associated with crying in therapy and surmised that the affective valence that may cause "neurotics" to cry in daily life outside of therapy differs from the affective valence leading to tears in therapy. They again suggest that a more positive affective tone may accompany tears in therapy. In a similar trend, the authors found that the trait of openness, which correlated most strongly with crying in therapy, only correlated with the subscale that measured crying in daily life due to positive situations and not at all with the subscale that measured crying in daily life due to negative situations, suggesting that those individuals who report the highest rates of crying in therapy are also most likely to cry in daily life due to positive situations.

While Blume-Marcovici et al.'s (2013) study, which looked at Big Five traits of personality, reported only equivocal findings regarding personality and crying in therapy, Tritt et al. (2015) asked clients in their study to rate their therapist in terms of "positive demeanor" traits (e.g., happy, firm, consistent) and "negative demeanor" traits (e.g., anxious, bored, angry) and found that the ways in which clients perceived their therapist's demeanor were directly related to the clients' experience of their therapist's tears. Those therapists who were rated as having a positive demeanor were reported to have looked close to tears or cried openly significantly more frequently, while those therapists who were perceived as having a negative demeanor were reported to have cried and ended a session more frequently. However, causality was not assessed. It could be that those therapists who were perceived positively were more likely to cry moderately because they are more happy, firm, and consistent, or it could be that their more moderate tears led to the client's perception of them as happy, firm, and consistent.

Personal Experience With Therapist Crying in Therapy

Brownlie's (2014) research with Australian psychologists found that those therapists who had experienced their own therapist tearing up or crying with them when they were in the client role were more prone to crying in therapy as therapists. It may be that these therapists felt permission to cry after having seen another therapist cry, or perhaps they found their therapist's tears helpful in some way, and therefore chose (however intentionally) to allow such an experience with their own clients. Alternatively, perhaps therapists who are prone to crying in therapy are simply more prone to seek out their own therapy, and thus have a greater chance of seeing their own therapist tear up.

Why Do Therapists Cry?

Since data, both anecdotal (Waldman, 1995) and quantitative (Blume-Marcovici et al., 2015), strongly refute the idea that therapists cry on purpose, other less volitional forces seem to be at work. Certainly some constitutional factors, such as "innate" crying tendency and personality, as discussed above, play a role in whether or not a therapist cries. But research suggests that there are relational dynamics and situation antecedents (e.g., session content) that contribute to therapists' tears as well.

Attachment and Caregiving

Mackie (2009), in a qualitative study of therapists' tears, identified three prototypes of therapists' tears based on distinct clusters of thoughts and emotions that occurred within therapists as their tears emerged, specific crying stimuli related to client presentation, and relational dynamics unfolding between the therapist and the client in the moment tears emerged. The three prototypes of tears are: (1) empathic tears, which emerge when the client is grieving the loss of a loved one; (2) caregiver tears, which emerge when therapists perceive their clients to be in a highly exposed and vulnerable state, such as when they disclose a story of abuse or trauma for the first time; and (3) proud-parent tears, which emerge when therapists perceive their clients to have achieved a crucial milestone in terms of their development and/or goals in therapy.

Mackie hypothesizes that each of these prototypes stimulates the therapist's attachment system into a state of high arousal (thereby prompting a tearful response), but that they do so in different ways. In the first instance, empathic tears are proposed to result from a process of empathic resonance. Losing a loved one is one of the most devastating attachment losses, and leads to an intense arousal of the attachment system (Bowlby, 1980). In witnessing their client's distress over such a loss, the therapists in Mackie's study described experiencing some of the same emotions of loss and grief that were apparent in their client, as if their own attachment system was humming alongside, or in resonance with, that of their client. Mackie described the other two prototypes of therapist's tears as emerging in the context of the caregiving dynamics unfolding within the therapeutic relationship. According to Bowlby (1982), as the organism matures, the attachment system grows into the attachment/caregiving system with the caregiving aspect being focused on, and responsive to, the needs of dependent others (i.e., infants). Mackie theorizes that "caregiver's tears" and "proud parent's tears" occur when this other half of the attachment system (i.e., the caregiving system) is stimulated into a state of high arousal. To illustrate, in the context of adult relationships, it has been proposed that the caregiving system has two primary goals. The first is to meet the other person's needs for protection and assistance when he or she is in difficulty, and the second goal is to foster growth and development in the relationship partner (Collins, Guichard, Ford, & Feeney, 2006). A therapist's "caregiver tears" appear to be consistent with the caregiving system's first goal of providing a safe haven for the relationship partner in his or her time of need (Bowlby, 1982). The therapist's experiences in instances of "proud parent's tears" seem consistent with the caregiving system's second core goal of fostering growth and development in the relationship partner.

Session Content

Each of Mackie's prototypes is associated with typical presenting material or clinical content areas: "empathic tears" are often associated with the clinical content of grief and loss, "caregiver tears" are often associated with the disclosure of abuse/trauma, and "proud parent tears" are often associated with client growth. In this, Mackie's research converges with existing data on which subjects or content areas in therapy sessions are most likely to cause a therapist to tear up. 't Lam and Vingerhoets (2016) reported that the most common content areas to accompany therapists' tears in therapy were clients' experiences of loss, especially the loss of a child or of a partner (i.e., "empathic tears"), emotional stories about a client's past, such as of abuse (i.e., "caregiver's tears"), as well as positive content areas such as the recovery of a client, feeling moved by the power of their client, or termination after a long period of successful therapy (i.e., "proud parent tears"). In Blume-Marcovici et al.'s (2015) qualitative study, the most common session topic in which therapist crying occurred was grief/loss (i.e., "empathic tears"), followed by trauma (i.e., "caregiver tears"), and termination of treatment (which we purport may be any of the three of Mackie's prototypes of tears, depending on the context). However, the authors noted that the session topics that accompanied crying varied greatly. In Waldman's qualitative study (1995), the majority of participants linked their crying in therapy to a current or past loss, or potential loss that was directly related to the client (i.e., "empathic tears"). Several participants also reported tears in therapy related to joyful or triumphant moments/ session topics or the therapist's sense of relief as a client described a positive change (i.e., "proud parent tears"). Based on these studies of session content related to therapists' tears, it appears that grief and loss, emotional discussions of abuse and trauma, witnessing profound growth in a client, and termination with a client (which can be experienced as a loss and/or as a positive moment in therapy) appear to be particularly common content areas in which therapist tearfulness may occur.

What Is the Impact on Treatment?

Research shows that therapists' tears most often have either a neutral or facilitative effect on treatment (Blume-Marcovici et al., 2013; Mackie, 2009; 't Lam & Vingerhoets, 2016; Tritt et al., 2015; Waldman, 1995). Of course, and of importance, therapists' tears can also have a harmful impact on treatment, though this seems to be rarer (Blume-Marcovici et al., 2013; 't Lam & Vingerhoets, 2016; Tritt et al., 2015; Waldman, 1995) and may be related to more intense or frequent crying (Brownlie, 2014) or crying that occurs before the therapeutic relationship has been established (Nelson, 2007). In short, research (described in detail below) shows that whether therapist crying is seen as valuable or harmful appears to depend on the overall context of the therapy and relationship between the therapist and client (Blume-Marcovici et al., 2013; Brownlie, 2014; Nelson, 2007; Tritt et al., 2015).

Three studies have investigated the impact of therapists' tears from the client's perspective (Pendleton, 2015; Tritt et al., 2015; Watson, 2015). Tritt et al. (2015) found both short- and long-term positive benefits of therapists' tears, depending on the client's perception of the therapist's demeanor. They note that the tears of a therapist had a positive impact on therapy if the therapist was seen as having an overall positive demeanor, with the greatest impact on the client's respect for the therapist, willingness to express emotions, and willingness to undertake therapy in the future. Conversely, if the client perceived the therapist to have a negative demeanor, the therapist's tears tended to have a negative impact, with the client being less willing to express emotions in therapy or to undertake future therapy.

Watson (2015) interviewed eight people in the United Kingdom, ages 25–45, on their experience(s) of seeing their therapist cry during a session. Her data showed that witnessing a therapist's tears was a highly individual experience for the client, with the implications of therapists' tears ranging from very positive to very negative. Regardless of how the client reacted, all participants felt that the moment of their therapist's tears was a pivotal and highly influential moment in treatment that impacted how they felt toward the therapist, the therapy relationship, and even themselves. When experienced positively, Watson's participants noted that their therapist's tears were validating, increased their sense of connection in the relationship, gave them permission to emote themselves, and allowed them to feel powerful in their ability to effect and matter to another person (i.e., the therapist). When experienced negatively, participants described feeling that their therapist's tears decreased their (needed) belief in the therapist's abilities, powers, intentionality, and professionalism, made the relationship feel more friendly than professional, and brought up conflicts around who should care for whom in the relationship.

Pendleton (2015) interviewed eight inpatient adolescents, aged 13–17 years, in a qualitative study of clients' perspectives on therapists' tears. Based on content analysis, the two major themes she reported were the (1) beneficial and (2) detrimental impact of tears. In the beneficial category, Pendleton found three major subthemes. First, she found that therapists' tears could foster a deeper therapeutic connection. Interestingly, this could be the case when the tears were other-oriented (i.e., related to the client's experience) or self-oriented (i.e., related to the therapist's experience), as in one positive instance in which a child client asked her therapist about a loss in his family and he teared up as he answered her question. A second subtheme was that therapists' tears marked a turning point in treatment, with a portion of Pendleton's informants reporting that once they saw their therapist cry, the work became deeper and progressed more quickly. A third subtheme was that therapists' tears were perceived by clients as a sign of courage and emotional bravery in the therapist, which in turn allowed the client to have the courage to be emotionally vulnerable. Pendleton also found three subthemes when informants discussed their detrimental experiences of therapists' tears. First, therapists' tears could cause a role reversal, making several of her adolescent informants question the dependability of their adult therapist. Second, therapists' tears could cause the client to withdraw from therapy, either emotionally or through terminating the treatment. These informants reported feeling that the therapist was emotionally weak, could not handle them and consequently they shared less in the treatment, or stopped the treatment altogether. The third subtheme was that therapists' tears could cause discomfort. These informants described the therapist trying to connect on a level that the client simply was not ready for.

From the therapist's perspective, 't Lam and Vingerhoets (2016) found that nearly half of all therapists who had cried in their study felt their tears had a positive effect on their clients in the short term and over a third purported that their tears also had a positive long-term effect. Research on therapists' understanding of the impact of their tears shows that, when viewed as positively impacting, therapists' tears can affirm to the client the therapist's ability to understand the client's distress and validate such distress (Blume-Marcovici et al., 2013; Mackie, 2009; Waldman, 1995), communicate genuineness and authenticity (Blume-Marcovici et al., 2013; Waldman, 1995), show the client that the therapist truly cares about him/her (Blume-Marcovici et al., 2013), facilitate the client's own ability to express affect (Blume-Marcovici et al., 2013; Waldman, 1995), model appropriate emotional expression (Blume-Marcovici et al., 2013), develop a more relaxed and trusting climate (Mackie, 2009), and strengthen the therapeutic rapport (Blume-Marcovici et al., 2013; Mackie, 2009; Waldman, 1995). Mackie (2009) noted that when therapists' tears fell within the prototype of caregiver's tears, they were most likely to be associated with a positive effect on the therapy by creating a sense of validation and support and strengthening the relationship. Therapists also report that their tears at times lead to new insights about their client, as was the case in 28% of the most recent crying episodes of the psychotherapists and trainees Blume-Marcovici et al. (2013) surveyed.

Therapists report the potential negative impact of their tears to be a fear on the client's part that the therapist will be overwhelmed by his/her own feelings (Blume-Marcovici et al., 2013; Waldman, 1995), that the therapist will not be able to help the client (Waldman, 1995), that the client will be burdened by the therapist's emotions (Blume-Marcovici et al., 2013; 't Lam & Vingerhoets, 2016), and that a role reversal may occur (Blume-Marcovici et al., 2013; Nelson, 2007). Some therapists report that therapist crying is simply unprofessional or even unethical ('t Lam & Vingerhoets, 2016). In order to minimize the potential of harm, therapists report it is necessary to maintain a client focus (Brownlie, 2014; Nelson, 2007).

It appears that whether or not a therapist discusses his/her tears may have a mediating effect on the impact of a therapist's tears. Blume-Marcovici et al. (2013) found that the 39% of their survey respondents who discussed their tears with their client were significantly more likely to report improvement in the relationship than those who did not discuss tears. However, they did not study what such discussions looked like, whether they were simple acknowledgments that the topic was moving or sad, or whether they were more indepth discussions about the therapeutic dynamic or the meaning of emotional expressions. Watson (2015) found that, among her participants (clients who had experienced their therapist cry in a session), there were mixed reactions to *not* discussing tears (of note, the ways in which therapists may have actually discussed their tears did not emerge as a major theme in the study). Those clients who tended to have a positive experience of their therapist's tears remarked that they appreciated that the therapist allowed silence around the tears, letting the tears speak for themselves. These clients liked that the therapist did not excuse or apologize for the tears. Others, especially the two participants for whom their therapist's tears were aversive, wished that the tears had been explained or explored further. These clients were left to worry that they had done something wrong to cause their therapist distress and described feeling guilty or to blame for something they did not quite understand. From this small sample, we may surmise that discussing tears is especially important in cases in which the therapist is concerned about the potential negative impact of his/her own tears, as a client-focused discussion may serve to bring to light and work through client concerns.

CONCLUSION

This chapter has reviewed research on therapists' tears in therapy. While the studies are few, and several are limited by small sample size, there are a number of trends that emerge regarding therapists' tears. Firstly, it seems that therapists' tears are a relatively common occurrence, by which we mean that, although tears do not tend to occur frequently (quite the opposite, as they tend to be rare), most therapists have cried in therapy. Secondly, it does not seem that therapists' tears are the catastrophic event that some therapists fear. While adverse impacts have been recorded, and are certainly important to consider, research suggests there are quite a few potential positive effects. It also seems that a client-centered discussion of therapists' tears with a client can ameliorate some of the risk of negative affects. There remains much to be learned about tears in therapy—both clients' and therapists'—and the ways in which such moments of emotional disclosure on the part of the therapist can influence, for better or worse, the larger course of treatment.

REFERENCES

Bindra, D. (1972). Weeping, a problem of many facets. *Bulletin of the British Psychological Society*, 25, 281–284.

Blume-Marcovici, A. C., Stolberg, R. A., & Khademi, M. (2013). Do therapists cry in therapy? The role of experience and other factors in therapists' tears. *Psychotherapy: Theory, Research, Practice, Training*, 50, 224–234.

Blume-Marcovici, A. C., Stolberg, R. A., & Khademi, M. (2015). Examining our tears: Therapists' accounts of crying in therapy. *American Journal of Psychotherapy*, 69(4), 399–421.

Borquist, A. (1906). Crying. *The American Journal of Psychology*, 17(April), 149–205.

Bowlby, J. (1980). *Attachment and loss: Loss, sadness and depression* (Vol. III). London: The Hogarth Press.

Bowlby, J. (1982). *Attachment and loss: Attachment* (2nd ed., Vol. 1). New York, NY: Basic Books.

Brownlie, M. R. (2014). *Uncharted 'tearitory': Mapping Australian therapist experiences, attitudes, and understandings of their in-session tears.* Unpublished master's thesis abstract. Monash University, Australia.

Bylsma, L. M., Vingerhoets, A. J. J. M., & Rottenberg, J. (2008). When is crying cathartic? An international study. *Journal of Social and Clinical Psychology*, 27(10), 1165–1187.

Collins, N., Guichard, A., Ford, M., & Feeney, B. (2006). Responding to need in intimate relationships: Normative processes and individual differences. In M. Mikulincer & G. Goodman (Eds.), *Dynamics of romantic love: Attachment, caregiving, and sex* (pp. 149–189). New York, NY: Guilford Press.

Cova, F., & Deonna, J. A. (2014). Being moved. *Philosophical Studies*, 169, 447–466.

Denckla, C. A., Fiori, K. L., & Vingerhoets, A. J. J. M. (2014). Development of the crying proneness scale: Associations among crying proneness, empathy, attachment, and age. *Journal of Personality Assessment, 96*, 619–631.

John, O. P., & Srivastava, S. (1999). The big five trait taxonomy: History, measurement, and theoretical perspectives. In L. A. Pervin & O. P. John (Eds.), *Handbook of personality: Theory and research* (pp. 102–138). New York, NY: Guilford Press.

Mackie, A. (2009). *When the therapist cries in psychotherapy: The meaning and impact of the therapist's tears.* Unpublished honours thesis. Australia: Swinburne University.

Nelson, J. K. (2007). Crying by the therapist. *Access: Your Link to the Clinical Social Work Association*, Summer, 9–17.

Pendleton, K. (2015). *Female adolescents' experience of their therapist crying in therapy.* Master's thesis. University of Kentucky: Theses and Dissertations, Family Sciences, Paper 24.

Pope, K. S., Tabachnick, B. G., & Keith-Spiegel, P. (1987). Ethics of practice: The beliefs and behaviors of psychologists as therapists. *American Psychologist, 42*, 993–1006.

Robinson, N., Hill, C. E., & Kivlighan, D. M. (2015). Crying as communication in psychotherapy: The influence of client and therapist attachment dimensions and client attachment to therapist on amount and type of crying. *Journal of Counseling Psychology, 62*(3), 379–392.

't Lam, C., & Vingerhoets, A. J. J. M. (2016). De tranen van de therapeut. [The tears of the therapist.] *De Psycholoog, 7*, 10–20.

Trezza, G. R., Hastrup, J. L., & Kim, S. E. (1988). *Clinicians' attitudes and beliefs about crying behavior.* Fifty-ninth Annual Meeting of the Eastern Psychological Association, Buffalo, NY.

Tritt, A., Kelly, J., & Waller, G. (2015). Patients' experiences of clinicians' crying during psychotherapy for eating disorders. *Psychotherapy, 52*(3), 373–380.

Vingerhoets, A. J. J. M., & Bylsma, L. M. (2016). The riddle of human emotional crying: A challenge for emotion researchers. *Emotion Review, 48*(3), 207–217.

Waldman, J. L. (1995). *Breakthrough or breakdown: When the psychotherapist cried during the therapy session.* Doctoral dissertation. Retrieved from Dissertation and Theses database. UMI No. 9536358.

Watson, A. (2015). *When therapists cry: Client's experience of witnessing therapist's tears. An interpretative phenomenological analysis.* Unpublished Honours dissertation. University of East London, London.

Williams, D. G., & Morris, G. H. (1996). Crying, weeping or tearfulness in British and Israeli adults. *British Journal of Psychology, 87*, 479–505.

CONSTRUCTS OF CRYING: UNDERSTANDING TEARS THROUGH THEORY

CHAPTER 3

THE FEELING IS MUTUAL: THERAPIST CRYING FROM AN ATTACHMENT/ CAREGIVING PERSPECTIVE

Judith Kay Nelson

> It is an everyday scene captured on video: a mother diapering a newborn infant. To the dismay of the audience (I have shown it countless times to students), the baby is tense, flailing and crying with a shrieking tone. If the audience pauses to look at the face of the mother (who it must be said is "causing" the baby to cry with this necessary task) or to listen to her sounds and words, it is clear that she is caught between completing her task as quickly as possible and soothing the baby's distress. At one point, she stops and leans over to enfold the baby in her warm body, nuzzling her little head, and saying, "Oh my god, oh my god, shh, shh," words of maternal distress uttered in a calm voice. Finally, she stands up and hurries to finish with the diaper change while the baby returns to shrieking. When it is over, the mother picks up the baby with a gentle, drawn out cheer, "Yea! Yea!" followed by a sweetly sympathetic, "Oh, my poor babe, yea, much better, ey?" As the baby quiets and settles on her shoulder, the camera catches the mother's face. We see her roll her eyes to the ceiling in a gesture of complete relief, smile, and give a small chuckle. At last, all is well for both mother and baby.
>
> (Spidell & Thalenberg, 2004)

This chapter begins by describing the attachment/caregiving system and how crying is an integral aspect of this system in infancy and beyond. The middle section shows how the attachment/caregiving system can be applied to understand crying—by client or therapist—in the therapeutic context. The final part discusses four prototypes of therapists' tears that can occur within the therapeutic attachment bond.

CRYING FROM AN ATTACHMENT/CAREGIVING PERSPECTIVE

Attachment behaviors are universal, inborn, and unlearned, and crying, a behavior present from birth, is at the top of the list, serving as it does to powerfully beckon the caregiver when the infant is negatively aroused, most significantly by separation from the caregiver. Crying is an unambiguous signal of negative arousal in the infant that creates corresponding negative arousal in the caregiver (Boukydis & Burgess, 1982; Donovan & Leavitt, 1985), calling for a caregiving response. In recent decades, attachment researchers have expanded Bowlby's (1969) original definition of attachment as an inborn behavior designed to bring about proximity to the caregiver to include attachment as the dyadic regulation of affect, a definition that might be applied to psychotherapy as well. Thus, in responding to infant cries, caregivers soothe and regulate not only the infant's negative arousal but also their own.

The attachment and caregiving systems are reciprocal—attachment behaviors trigger caregiving behaviors—in the parent–infant relationship and in close relationships throughout life, including the therapeutic relationship. The process, mutual and intersubjective from the outset, results from the intertwining of two nervous systems so that there is reciprocity of both affect arousal and affect regulation. Contributions from neurobiological studies of attachment reinforce the idea that individuals rapidly and subliminally transmit affect through facial expressions, including tearing up and crying, bodily posture, tone of voice, and gaze, and that affect is indeed mutually aroused and mutually regulated (Schore, 2003). Musical analogies to this biologically based interconnection come to mind: resonance, improvisation, rhythmic synchronization, or entrainment.

The beckoning, attachment-building power of infant crying and the way in which it viscerally evokes caregiving responses is a template for crying throughout life. Adult crying, too, is an attachment behavior that triggers caregiving behavior. A stranger crying on the steps of the post office, a friend sharing a diagnosis of breast cancer, or a client bereaved at the loss of a parent all alert potential caregivers to the pain of loss and trigger powerful urges to offer caregiving help or comfort. Negative arousal in the crier disturbs a potential caregiver, analogous to the way that infant crying does with a parent. An attachment/caregiving framework provides a basis for bringing some of that ephemeral process to consciousness.

Crying, Separation, and Grief

The default reason for crying in infancy is at separation from the caregiver, and for adults at the death of a close loved one (Bowlby, 1960, 1961). Separation and loss are the key precipitants for tears throughout life. In infancy, the primary threat is to the loss of life, as the infant is unable to survive in the absence of a caregiver. Losses in adult life, though they may feel equally life-threatening, go beyond loss by death to include the "deaths" or endings of everyday life such as divorce, break-up, empty nest, retirement, or relocation, or losses that are symbolic, threatened, fantasized, or imagined. Repeatedly, the clichéd lines, "If you leave me I will cry; If you leave me I will die," link loss of a lover and death.

Grief is the process set in motion when separations and losses occur. Regardless of the source or severity, a loss may lead to a grief reaction parallel to those that occur with death or separation from the caregiver. Grief reactions, no matter the precipitant, sometimes trigger the attachment behavior of crying—an appeal for a caregiving response. When we grieve, we sometimes cry, but when we cry it almost always represents a grief reaction (Nelson, 2005).

While studying infants placed in war nurseries in England during World War II, Bowlby (1960, 1980) identified three stages of grief: protest, despair, and detachment. Subsequently, he observed that the responses of adults to the loss of a close loved one parallel those of an infant separated from the caregiver (Bowlby, 1961). Bowlby mentioned in passing the types of crying that accompanied protest, despair, and detachment in the infants separated from their caregivers in the nurseries. Protest crying was a loud, high-energy cry, an emergency signal designed to bring about a speedy end to the separation. If there was no reunion and no consistent substitute caregiver, the infant would go into a state of despair, where the crying was more of a low wail. Finally, if the separation continued indefinitely, the child would go into a detached, non-crying silent state.

Looking at the parallels between adult grief and infant grief, I theorized that the quality of adult crying might also change in relationship to each stage of grief (Nelson, 2005). Adult crying could then be classified according to the stage of grief to which it corresponds, with protest crying being of high intensity, designed to undo or avoid a loss, and crying in despair, a quiet weeping that represents surrender to the reality of a loss. Detached tearlessness, a silent, withdrawn depression in response to a loss, would correspond to an infant's life-threatening detachment following permanent separation from a caregiver.

Crying and Attachment Style

In understanding the attachment/caregiving elements of crying in therapy—by the therapist or by the client—it is important to recognize both the stage of grief to which the crying corresponds and the attachment style of the crier and the caregiver (Robinson, Hill, & Kivlighan, 2015). Attachment style, so named by Ainsworth (1967), an early attachment researcher, is what Bowlby (1969) termed the "internal working model of attachment" (p. 80). The individual's attachment style is based on early attachment and caregiving experiences, and represents a neurobiological template for close relationships, affect arousal, and affect regulation throughout life (Mikulincer & Shaver, 2007). From neurobiological research, we now understand that attachment style represents the impact on the infant's developing brain and nervous system of repeated cycles of arousal, attunement/misattunement, and regulation between infant and caregiver (Schore, 2003). The infant's nervous system constellates its affect-regulating strategies around these experiences in the early years of life to form what we call attachment style.

Based on the huge body of attachment-style research, we have learned that secure attachment results from consistent, attuned, and reliable caregiver responses to affect arousal, both negative and positive (Nelson, 2012; Schore, 2003). Insecure attachment styles in adults include preoccupied or dismissing. People with preoccupied attachment styles typically have experienced inconsistent, highly reactive, or overly smothering caregiving early in life, while the dismissing style is linked to excesses of early independence training and underresponse on the part of the caregiver to the infant's affect arousal.

Though secure attachment with an attuned and responsive caregiver is the primary strategy with which infants are born, some infants must adapt by using secondary strategies to accommodate overly anxious, inconsistent, or neglectful caregivers. When caregivers are abusive, fearful of the infant, or severely depressed or neglectful, no adaptive strategy is possible, resulting in a tendency toward dissociation in response to negative arousal, and to conflicting patterns of arousal and regulation, known as disorganized attachment (Main & Solomon, 1990).

Crying is our first attachment behavior and constitutes our first intersubjective experience. Over time, the successes and failures at beckoning caregivers by crying and the appropriateness, effectiveness, and promptness of their responses contribute to the establishment and maintenance of the attachment bond as well as to its quality, whether secure, preoccupied, dismissing, or disorganized.

CRYING IN THE CONTEXT OF THE THERAPEUTIC ATTACHMENT BOND

As described above, when caregivers soothe and regulate a crying infant, they also soothe their own negative arousal. Likewise, a client's affect in therapy may produce negative arousal in the therapist—discomfort, sadness, anxiety—that he/she soothes and regulates as an important part of the caregiving process. Indeed, Stolorow and Atwood (1992) write that "proper domain of psychoanalytic inquiry is not the isolated individual mind, but the larger system created by the mutual interplay between the subjective worlds of patient and analyst, or of child and caregiver" (p. 1). This intersubjective view of the therapeutic relationship was launched in large part by research that showed infants and parents to be dynamic partners in a mutually regulating attachment and caregiving relationship (Beebe, Lachmann, & Jaffe, 1997; Stern, 1985). Using the model of the attachment/caregiving system to understand crying in therapy—by either the client or the therapist—helps to shed light on the many nuances of the intersubjective interaction that crying in therapy represents. Indeed, from an intersubjective attachment/caregiving standpoint, the distinction between the person shedding the tears and the non-crier (or mutual crier) becomes increasingly blurred. By keeping the attachment/caregiving theoretical model in mind, the psychotherapist can contextualize the therapy relationship within the attachment histories of both parties (Robinson, Hill, & Kivlighan, 2015), as well as more consciously monitor affect arousal, including crying by either partner, and the attunements and misattunements that may result. Utilizing this model can help the therapist understand confusing countertransference responses that may trigger the therapist's crying or lead to unexplained or unwelcome reactions to crying by the client. This model can also help us to formulate important guidelines for when a therapist should restrain from crying and why crying by the therapist sometimes helps and sometimes interferes.

Loss is a primary theme for virtually every client who comes for therapy. Such losses vary widely in time, from childhood to present day or to anticipation of future loss; in intensity, from large to small; and in social spheres ranging from intimate relationships, to athletic, academic, or professional ones. Tears sometimes accompany grief, but whenever tears do appear, the vast majority of the time it is due to grief over a loss (Nelson, 2005). The small remaining experiences of crying represent either physiologically based crying (for example, strokes, medication side-effects, endocrine disorders) or true tears of joy and connection, the other side of loss.

Therapists, too, have losses, alongside those of our clients. In general, it is the client whose attachment system is activated, thereby engaging the therapist's caregiving system. However, it is inevitable that the therapist's own attachment behaviors may be activated from time to time, even as we are functioning fully in our role as professional caregivers. Attachment and caregiving are reciprocal systems that represent the intertwining of the affective lives of the partners in the therapeutic dyad. As parents experience the infant's negative arousal and become negatively aroused themselves, so do therapists experience the pain and grief of their client's losses, resulting at times in sharing their pain, identifying with it, or triggering the therapist's own loss and grief. The result is that sometimes therapists cry with our clients or instead of our clients—over their losses, our losses, or some immeasurable mixture of the two.

An attachment/caregiving approach to understanding crying in the clinical hour—by either party—requires attuning to three key principles. They are: the stage of grief, attachment styles (of client and therapist), and the state of the therapeutic attachment bond.

The Stage of Grief

Protest

Protest grief in adulthood is the cry of "no" in response to a loss that urges the caregiver/therapist to do something to prevent or undo the loss, as protest crying in infancy serves as an emergency signal to bring the caregiver back to the child. Other than in the aftermath of a traumatic loss, protest crying comes across as demanding, blaming, angry, dissatisfied, or devaluing of the caregiver. Protest crying is more likely to evoke feelings of apathy, irritation, guilt, or a loss of confidence rather than empathy in the therapist caregiver. Protest criers are not open to empathic caregiving; they simply want action to avert or undo or in some way compensate for their loss.

Maintaining an intersubjective balance in the face of protest grief is challenging and requires a great deal of skill and forbearance. I recall, for example, a client crying in protest grief over my pending vacation. Tearfully, she attacked me, saying, "You travel too much! You know my fears of abandonment and how my parents left me with strangers. This is abusive; I'm going to find another therapist." She succeeded in arousing corresponding negative affect in me, but it was a mixture of anxiety, guilt, and irritation. In effect she was saying, "You are making me cry by threatening this loss," which was literally true, and I acknowledged it empathically. I then attempted to soothe her by explaining why I needed to travel and going over the arrangements for her care in my absence. As I spoke to her, I, too, was calmed. Regulating her affect regulated mine as well.

If a therapist does cry in response to protest grief, the outcome is almost certainly doomed without a lot of skillful processing by the therapist. One such example came to me from a new client who reported that she had become dissatisfied with her previous therapy and presented some of her complaints to the therapist. When she confronted her, the therapist burst into tears without explaining why. The client was alarmed, confused, and angry at the therapist's protesting response (the reasons for it were not disclosed or discussed) and she terminated. Having the therapist's attachment system activated in response to her protest made the client feel insecure with the therapeutic caregiver and even more anxious about getting the help she wanted.

Despair

This stage of grief represents surrender to the reality of a loss. Like the intermittently crying infant slumped in the corner of the crib, the adult has given up hope of the loss being restored or averted. This is the type of crying that evokes the strongest desire in the caregiver to connect and comfort the crier. As a result, it is this type of crying where healing is most likely to occur.

Despair is also the type of grief most likely to elicit crying by the therapist. Certainly the client's narrative about a loss can be evocative, but his or her posture, gaze, and tone of voice also speak volumes to our implicit, procedural brains. The therapist may be similarly moved to tears, crying along with the client, identifying through a similar personal loss, or purely from empathy. Other clients speak in a flat, tearless tone while the therapist is the one who cries. A number of experienced therapists I interviewed cited examples of such empathic crying when they shed tears for a client before he or she was able to do so—a perfect example of a mutual, intersubjective attachment/caregiving moment (Nelson, 2005).

Detachment

Infants go into shut-down mode when there is no end to the separation, and some adults do so as well. Not only do they inhibit crying, but they also withdraw into an isolated depression, shutting out all attempts at caregiving.

Detached adults do not typically come to therapy voluntarily unless blindsided by unexpected grief at the loss of a mate or job. In any case, crying creates extreme discomfort for them, and potential caregivers, including the therapist, are held at bay, sometimes coldly, sometimes angrily, and sometimes in a manner as flat as their overall affect. As in infancy, detachment can also be a life-threatening form of grief for adults who may stop eating or become suicidal.

While therapists are far more likely to feel ineffective, frustrated, blamed, or even irritated than to tear up in the face of detachment, it is possible that an interpersonal chord could nonetheless be struck, resulting in a therapist crying. If so, the likelihood of misinterpretation by the detached client is high, meaning that the therapist should quickly check out how the client is perceiving the therapist's tears. If the client is not able or willing to be forthcoming, the therapist can help to fill in the blanks by explaining the source of her tears and the feelings that prompted them. It would not be safe to assume that the client would experience the tears as empathic or sympathetic.

Attachment Style

As described earlier, attachment style forms the neurobiological template for affect arousal (crying) and affection regulation (caregiving). The attachment styles of client and therapist, therefore, come into play with experiences of crying by either party (Robinson, Hill, & Kivlighan, 2015). For example, differences in attachment style—of therapist as well as client—relate to frequency and type of crying (Robinson et al., 2015), ease and intensity of arousal or showing vulnerability, expectations for appropriate and effective attunement, and the ability to trust in and rely upon a caregiver to participate in affect regulation. Thus, an understanding of the theory and research related to attachment styles has deep relevance for understanding the therapeutic process and relationship (Cassidy & Shaver, 2008; Mikulincer & Shaver, 2007; Schore 2003).

Secure Attachment

Securely attached people are those most comfortable with crying, their own and that of others, though that does not necessarily mean that they cry more (Robinson et al., 2015). They have developed a sense of confidence that distress can be revealed to caregivers with the expectation that it will be understood and regulated. In addition, securely attached people are able to rely on internalized caregivers for self-regulation. This is not to say that securely attached people have not experienced misattunements or that their comfort with crying is complete. Social mores and judgments about tears may also be internalized, and even the most securely attached person—client or therapist—may apologize for crying, defend against it, or prefer to cry in solitude.

Preoccupied Attachment

Preoccupied adults, having grown up insecure about whether caregivers will respond to crying appeals in an attuned or effective manner, are quick to activate attachment behaviors such as crying in order to attract caregiving, while simultaneously having little confidence that a caregiver can effectively regulate their arousal. Their fallback belief is that the caregiver will ignore or overreact, leaving them to dangle alone and unsoothed. Until a more secure therapeutic attachment bond is established, protest grief is a common presentation.

Dismissing Attachment

The attachment/caregiving profile of a person who is dismissing rotates around an internal working model of independence, self-regulation, and a tendency to defensively deactivate the attachment system. Because there is no experience or expectation of a caregiver response built in from early life, crying is squelched and considered intrusive and unwelcome. Grief may be expressed directly or indirectly in angry protests, humor, or intellectualizing, with tears emerging only when overwhelming grief breaks through their defensive deactivation or after they have begun to experience earned security in the context of the therapeutic attachment bond.

The State of the Therapeutic Attachment Bond

Over the course of a treatment relationship, the type of crying may change, reflecting the level of security the client feels with the therapist. Attuning to the frequency of tears, whether they are tears of protest, despair, or the non-crying that accompanies withdrawn detachment, gives the therapist a guide to the internal working models of attachment operating within the therapeutic relationship. The therapist's inclination or disinclination to cry in response to the client's pain, grief, and loss will be one way to gauge the client's level of attachment security with the therapist.

For example, in the early phases of working with a withdrawn, detached person, the therapist may actually be shedding tears of grief that has not been acknowledged or even felt by the client. At a later stage, however, the client may move into protest grief, perhaps directed at the therapist, and the therapist may feel defensive or irritated rather than carrying the earlier, unexpressed grief. While it seems paradoxical, this is a move toward greater security in the therapeutic relationship. In yet another later phase, as the client moves toward earned secure attachment and is able to cry in despair, the therapist may again feel the urge to cry in empathy.

THERAPIST CRYING IN THE CLINICAL HOUR

In earlier writing (Nelson, 2005, 2007), I outlined some common types of crying by the therapist identified through surveys of experienced therapists, conversations with colleagues, and personal experience. The types are: crying as connection; crying when the therapist is undergoing a personal, acute grief reaction; and crying at termination. I discuss each type below, and have added a section on crying at retirement as I have found—based on personal experience and discussions with other professionals—that terminations at retirement may represent an amalgam of these three types of therapists' tears.

Crying as Connection

A number of therapists report this type of crying to be a form of empathic attunement to the client and see it as an extension of their caregiving function rather than an activation of their attachment system. In a number of the examples I collected, however, therapists clearly identified an intersubjective element, recognizing that their crying was linked to some overlap between the client's loss and an undisclosed loss of the therapist's.

A number of the responses to my survey came from therapists reflecting back on their own therapist crying in a session. Several recalled it as one of the most meaningful experiences in the therapeutic relationship, though two made qualifications. One said that the crying had taken place five years into the work, but that had it occurred earlier, she would have assumed that her pain was too overwhelming for the therapist. Another reported a changing view as she came to know some details about her therapist's life. When he originally cried with her over the loss of her parents in childhood, she was moved and did indeed feel a deepened connection. Later, however, when she learned that he had also lost his parents at an early age, she felt the experience much diluted, almost tainted, by the fact that his tears were also about his grief, and not solely about hers.

While a therapist crying in this way may represent to the therapist the deepest form of connection with the client, the client may misinterpret it as the therapist's attachment behavior rather than a caregiving one. In a workshop I led recently, a participant recounted having teared up as her client described losing her mother as a young girl. The therapist teared up and acknowledged that she, too, had lost her mother at about the same age. The client got upset at the intrusion of the therapist's grief and complained to the student's supervisor, saying that the therapist had "burst into tears" (not the therapist's recollection at all). The supervisor shared the complaint with other members of the clinical team and these colleagues joined forces in being extremely judgmental and condemning of the therapist's behavior. This example cries out, as it were, for more open and thoughtful discussion about crying by the therapist in training programs. Being able to return and process such an experience with the client, as with any other inadvertent break in empathy, would have been foreclosed had the student not been mature enough to persist in explaining herself in the face of such lack of support and understanding from her colleagues.

Crying During an Acute Grief Reaction

There are no guidelines for how soon a therapist should go back to work after the loss of a close loved one. Nonetheless, it can be assumed that for at least some months after a painful loss a bereaved therapist will be in the throes of grief with increased vulnerability to crying during therapy. Some unexpected overlap or association in a session may unleash tears that may appear intense or uncharacteristic to the client. In fact, I happened to know the therapist described above who burst into tears when her client confronted her with her dissatisfaction with the therapy, and I knew that she had chosen to return to work just several days after the loss of her child. Unfortunately, the therapist chose not to disclose her loss to her clients so that her crying could be understood in context. There are, however, also numerous examples of therapists experiencing severe grief reactions who do share the fact of their loss with their clients and who find that doing so, even when the therapist might cry, deepens the connection.

Crying at Termination

Three of the four times I cried throughout my 40 years as a psychotherapist (aside from crying during my retirement process, which I will discuss below) were at unexpected and painful terminations. Two of them were with children, which made my intersubjective vulnerability all the more intense. The first was a 12-year-old girl who had to leave town abruptly to go live with relatives because her custodial parent was murdered. The other was with a teenager whose parents ran out of patience and decided to send her away to school. Neither client cried and I feared that my doing so would further upset them. However, the first girl took my tears to mean what they were: that I was attached to her and would feel her loss. It represented our connection and had so much meaning that years later she came back to town to check in with the detective handling her parent's case and called me. The second girl told me, when I asked how she felt about my crying, that of all the people she had told she was leaving, I was the only one who cried. To her it was a clear sign of how much I cared about her and would miss her—caregiving and attachment behavior rolled into one.

My third experience of termination tears was more complex and conflicted. A young woman in her 30s was terminating prematurely, declaring that she had gotten what she had come for, though my sense was that she was fleeing the work still to be done. I unsuccessfully fought tears in one session as she discussed her decision and I realized I needed to get consultation. I think now that my crying represented tears of protest—my attempt to prevent or undo her decision about the separation/termination. Because of the complex ways in which protest crying can be used to control others or make them feel guilty, however, it was both unwise and ineffectual. I knew I needed to control my tears in order to find enough caregiving neutrality to help her process her feelings about the proposed ending.

Crying at Retirement

If there are no guidelines about when to return to work after an acute grief reaction, there are certainly no rules about how to negotiate multiple terminations during a retirement process. When I retired after almost 40 years of psychotherapy practice, I announced my retirement one to two years ahead depending on the client. As another retiring colleague stated, however, "The client may need one year's notice, but so does the therapist." Her remark points to the deeply intersubjective nature of retirement terminations. The therapist needs time to process endings in multiple relationships, and to end a phase of life and give up a professional identity. In other words, as another colleague who retired recently said, "Be prepared for a lot of tears." She did not specify whose tears she was referring to, but from experience, I can attest to the fact that mine were as much a part of the equation as were my clients'. When a therapist closes a practice, the usual mutuality of the ending is intensified.

In addition, retirement precludes the usual assumption—spoken or unspoken—that the client could decide to return in the future.

In my experience, following months of tearless processing, it was in the final session when the actual goodbyes were spoken that the tears began to flow. Even in writing that sentence now, I feel a lump in my throat. Two examples stand out, and both were with young adult women (early 20s) who had suffered much trauma and loss in their lives, in one case the recent loss of a parent. The journey we had shared as we built bridges from traumatic childhoods to mature adult life was too all-encompassing for words. I had been part of their growth, but I had grown, too, in response to their suffering and their courage. One, a writer, was eloquent as she tried to express the meaning of our relationship and we both quietly wept throughout. The other was the only client who, upon hearing of my retirement, brightened and said, "I'm so happy for you!" with a sincerity and generosity that were more than defense against her pain. For our last session, she came bearing a huge bouquet of flowers, which even now makes me weep. The flowers were both funereal and celebratory, though my affect matched the former more than the latter.

Things were much less straightforward, however, with several clients I had been seeing for barely two years following the death of their long-term therapist, my close friend and office partner. In this instance, the clients and I shared a mutual acute grief reaction over the loss of a long-term therapist and a beloved friend. Now they were losing me, and their connection to the office building. In all three instances, the pain of their grief was deep and they knew I shared in their loss, though at no point did my tears threaten to erupt. It was burdensome to have to compartmentalize my grief, but it also felt necessary that I preserve my affect-regulating, caregiving function for them. I needed to endure so that they could endure. Mine was an intersubjective, caregiving decision.

CONCLUSION AND RECOMMENDATIONS

Attachment and caregiving forces are continually at work in the therapeutic relationship, drawing on the therapist's procedural knowledge of affect arousal, attunement, and regulation. Having a sense of one's own attachment style, and the associated affect arousal and regulation patterns, aids the therapist in understanding these complex dynamics. When all is going smoothly, it is not necessary to take the step of making the implicit explicit, but when misattunements or enactments intrude around crying by either party, an attachment/caregiving perspective is crucial for making conscious sense of the dynamics and for processing them with the client.

A recent research study testing some aspects of an attachment/caregiving perspective on crying in the clinical hour suggests that, in order to understand the meaning of crying in the therapeutic relationship, therapists need to attend to the overall amount of client crying, the type of crying, their own and their client's attachment style, and the client's attachment to the therapist. Further, they suggest that therapists be "attentive to their own attachment needs," which points to the fact that therapists also need caregiving in their lives (Robinson, Hill, & Kivlighan, 2015, p. 390). Therapists must maintain a high level of self-awareness regarding our own attachment needs and style so as not to get our clients to do our crying for us or unduly serve as our caregivers. We need to know our patterns well in order to sort through the intersubjective tangle of arousal and regulation. By keeping attachment and caregiving systems at the forefront, we can understand, welcome, process, and integrate the crying by either partner that occurs in the context of the therapeutic attachment/caregiving relationship.

REFERENCES

Ainsworth, M. (1967). *Infancy in Uganda: Infant care and the growth of love.* Baltimore, MD: Johns Hopkins University Press.

Beebe, B., Lachmann, F., & Jaffe, J. (1997). Mother–infant interaction structures and pre-symbolic self- and object representations. *Psychoanalytic Dialogues,* 7(2), 133–182.

Boukydis, C., & Burgess, R. (1982). Adult physiological response to infant cries: Effects of temperament of infant, parental status and gender. *Child Development,* 53, 1291–1298.

Bowlby, J. (1960). Grief and mourning in infancy and childhood. *Psychoanalytic Study of the Child,* 15(1), 9–52.

Bowlby, J. (1961). Processes of mourning. *The International Journal of Psychoanalysis,* 42(4–5), 317–339.

Bowlby, J. (1969). *Attachment.* New York, NY: Basic Books.

Bowlby, J. (1980). *Attachment and loss.* New York, NY: Basic Books.

Cassidy, J., & Shaver, P. (2008). *Handbook of attachment: Theory, research, and clinical application.* New York, NY: Guilford Press.

Donovan, W., & Leavitt, L. (1985). Physiology and behavior: Parents' response to the infant cry. In B. M. Lester & C. F. Boukydis (Eds.), *Infant crying: Theoretical and research perspectives* (pp. 241–259). New York, NY: Plenum Press.

Main, M., & Solomon, J. (1990). Procedures for identifying infants as disorganized/disoriented during the Ainsworth Strange Situation. In M. C. Greenberg (Ed.), *Attachment in the preschool years: Theory, research and intervention* (pp. 121–160). Chicago, IL: University of Chicago Press.

Mikulincer, M., & Shaver, P. R. (2007). *Attachment in adulthood: Structure, dynamics, and change.* New York, NY: Guilford Press.

Nelson, J. (2005). *Seeing through tears: Crying and attachment.* New York, NY: Routledge.

Nelson, J. K. (2007, January). When therapists cry. (J. Rosenfeld, Ed.) *Clinical Update, XXXVI* (6), pp. 1, 10, 12, 20.

Nelson, J. K. (2012). *What made Freud laugh: An attachment perspective on laughter.* New York, NY: Routledge.

Robinson, N., Hill, C., & Kivlighan, D. (2015). Crying as communication in psychotherapy: The influence of client and therapist attachment dimensions and client attachment to therapist on amount and type of crying. *Journal of Counseling Psychology, 62*(3), 379–392.

Schore, A. N. (2003). *Affect regulation and the repair of the self.* New York, NY: W.W. Norton.

Spidell, K. (Producer) & Thalenberg, E. (Director) (2004). *The baby human: Geniuses in diapers.* Canada: Ellis Vision Production in Association with Discovery Health Channel and Discovery Health Channel Canada.

Stern, D. N. (1985). *The interpersonal world of the infant: A view from psychoanalysis and developmental psychology.* New York, NY: Basic Books.

Stolorow, R., & Atwood, G. (1992). *Contexts of being: The intersubjective foundations of psychological life.* Hillsdale, NJ: The Analytic Press.

CHAPTER 4

AN EYE-OPENING EYE INFECTION: TREATING THERAPISTS' TEARS AS SELF-DISCLOSURE

Andrea Bloomgarden

> *Last year I had an eye infection that was causing my right eye to tear unexpectedly at any moment. While this was an inconvenience in many aspects of my life, I felt particularly self-conscious around my clients; I did not want them to think that I was crying at random in their sessions as they watched me wipe my eye. I had joked with my eye doctor that she had better fix my eye soon or my practice was going to suffer. We laughed together about my occupational hazard. I began announcing what was going on at the beginning of my sessions to prevent any misinterpretations. "My eye is tearing from an eye infection—I didn't want you to think I was crying or anything," I'd say, grabbing a tissue.*
>
> *"That's exactly it!" my client, Emily,[1] proclaimed, seeming suddenly energized by an insight. "Why wouldn't you just cry?"*
>
> *This was not the reaction I had expected.*

In this chapter, I will examine therapists' tears as a form of therapist self-disclosure. First, I will discuss how therapists' tears fit in the context of current self-disclosure literature. I will then review a model for keeping therapist self-disclosure therapeutic and apply this model to therapists' tears, as well as discuss how to balance client preferences with clinical wisdom. Once we have established the groundwork on tears within the self-disclosure literature, I will return to Emily's case, and introduce the case of Katie, in order to illustrate several of the myriad ways in which tears as self-disclosure may occur in the clinical setting.

THERAPIST SELF-DISCLOSURE

Therapists' Tears as a Form of Therapist Self-Disclosure

Crying is the least controlled and most authentic form of self-disclosure. Whether our eyes well up with tears or tears run down our cheeks, crying is an act of vulnerability—and humanity. As therapists we are in the sometimes difficult position of holding space for our clients. Is hiding our genuine emotions necessarily the best way to do that? Is it possible that, for some of our clients, our blunted, suppressed, or antiseptic emotional responses could actually be harmful?

Thoughtful therapist self-disclosure has been gradually moving away from its negative stereotype, and has been claiming its rightful place as a useful technique and important aspect of effective therapy, among a wide range of psychotherapeutic schools of thought (e.g., Aron, 1996; Baldwin, 2000; Bloomgarden & Mennuti, 2009; Brown, 1994; Farber, 2006; Hill & Knox, 2002; Kramer, 2000; Linehan, 1993; Maroda, 2004; Miller & Striver, 1997; Norcross, 2002; Rogers, 1989; Shapiro, 1995; Stricker & Fisher, 1990; Wachtel, 2008; Walker, 2004; Yalom, 2002; Zur, 2007a, 2007b). When therapists intentionally share something about themselves in a well-timed and attuned way, it can be normalizing, validating, or hope-inspiring. It can also be educational, teaching clients something relevant to their lives by using a personal example. On the other hand, there is valid concern when therapist self-disclosure is used carelessly, too frequently, or without awareness of its effect on the relationship. At worst, the therapy relationship might become indistinguishable from a social relationship, where the frame of therapy is lost and the client's reason for coming to therapy is all but ignored. The relationship can become ineffective, dysfunctional, or even harmful.

In the literature on therapist self-disclosure, many authors have discussed distinctions between types of therapist self-disclosure (e.g., Hill & Knox, 2002; Knox, Hess, Peterson, & Hill, 1997; Zur, 2009) and several concepts are relevant here. Most of the time, when we talk about self-disclosure, we are actually talking about *self-revealing self-disclosures* (also called *self-disclosing self-disclosures*). These are *factual* disclosures about ourselves, usually made with a therapeutic purpose in mind. By contrast, we self-disclose our *emotional reactions* to our clients through words, body language, and facial expression. In the literature, this has been called *self-involving self-disclosure*, as well as *immediacy*, that is, disclosing our feelings with the client in the moment. Crying with, for, or in response to our clients is usually a self-involving self-disclosure, conveying something we feel about our clients in the moment. It could also be a self-revealing one if we cry as we speak about something going on in our own life.

When tears are self-involving self-disclosure, the next question is whether they are *intentional* or *unintentional* (also referred to as *deliberate* or *non-deliberate self-disclosure*; Zur, 2009; Zur, Williams, Lehavot, & Knapp, 2009). In some cases, we may believe that allowing ourselves to cry with clients will convey an important message to them, and at such times, when the urge is there, we may choose to allow tears to come. In these moments, because we are choosing to share an emotional truth rather than holding it back, our tearful self-disclosure is intentional, even though crying is less in our control than a verbal disclosure. In other cases, tears may well up completely unexpectedly, representing an unintentional, even involuntary, self-disclosure. Although not initially intentional, our choice to discuss what has happened (both our experience of our tears and, perhaps more importantly, our client's reactions to our tears) moves us into the territory of intentional self-disclosure. In this sense, we treat therapists' tears as therapist self-disclosure by either intentionally allowing our tears, or by being curious about the effect of our tears upon the relationship through an intentional discussion about our (intentional or unintentional) tears.

Keeping Therapist Self-Disclosure Therapeutic

David Treadway provides a useful set of guidelines on self-disclosure (Treadway, 2009). He suggests that to keep self-disclosure from being a pointless self-indulgence, we should think through decisions in the following way:

1. Hypothesis. Have a hypothesis about how a particular disclosure might be helpful in the context of the session, in the present moment. *What is happening right now, and is it working or does something need to shift?*
2. Goal. What are we working on in therapy? There are broader, overarching, longer-term goals, and smaller, more immediate goals in any given session. An awareness of the therapy goals helps the therapist evaluate

whether or not the session is going well. *Is the session on track in terms of what I'm trying to achieve with this client today or does something need to shift?*
3. Strategies. Once we have a sense of the here-and-now experience in the room and its alignment (or misalignment) with therapy goals, we must choose an appropriate intervention. This is where we may consider self-disclosure. Whether we choose to share a fact, a feeling, a story, or tears, we are responding to what is going on in the room and making a choice about our next move, a choice that is ideally congruent with short- and long-term therapy goals. In the case of tears, this includes having a hypothesis about how the therapist's tears will be received in the moment. If we consider our clients' views about crying and their own relationship with crying, we may have some clues about how they will respond. *Will our tears potentially enhance or distract from therapy goals?* Depending on our clients' unique histories, they could have any number of interpretations of our tears (i.e., as validating, distracting, caring, weak), any of which may be helpful or unhelpful to their goals in therapy.
4. Outcome. After a self-disclosure, what happens next? *Did our disclosure seem to have the intended effect? Did the conversation become more productive? Did our client open up or shut down? Did the disclosure derail the session in a way that was not what we hoped for?* After a disclosure of any kind, be it tears or words, it is good practice to inquire about how it landed with the client—i.e., "What was it like for you that I got teary when you told me that?" This way, the client has permission to give honest feedback. When I have posed this exact question to clients regarding my tears, I have heard responses as varied as *"your tears were validating because no one has ever acted like it was a big deal before"* to *"you getting emotional made me feel unsafe because you should be taking care of me, not the other way around."* In the latter case, my tears were clearly not well received, but they did open up an important discussion about the life circumstances that led my client to feel this way. In this specific example, my client's parents had been neglectful, so she yearned for a parental figure who was strong for her all of the time. She experienced my expression of genuine emotion as me "falling apart" and that made her feel unsafe. While the rupture my tears caused was uncomfortable for us both, our discussion about my tears led to important insights in our work. Had I not inquired about her reaction, my tears may have led to an impasse in our relationship.

While these guidelines propose a lot to contemplate in any given moment, practicing with each of our clients helps us to know them better and to inform our future decisions around self-disclosure. Eventually, this process becomes instinctual, and we form a way of working with each client with attuned degrees of self-disclosure best suited to that relationship.

Balancing Client Preferences With Clinical Wisdom

Clients vary greatly in their preferences about therapist self-disclosure. Some clients feel grounded by a sense that there is a real person in the room with them, genuinely caring, transparently showing their emotional reactions, and sometimes discussing examples from their life. For them, therapist self-disclosure balances the power in the room and, only with this more equal status, do such clients feel comfortable being themselves. These clients are more likely to welcome a therapist's tears. Some clients feel precisely the opposite, and yearn for a space where they do not have to be concerned with their therapist's feelings or take care of their therapist in any way; perhaps therapy is the one place where they can be undistractedly self-focused and they need such a space. Thinking about their therapist as a person with emotions feels like a burden for these clients. Likewise, a therapist's tears, or too much disclosure of any kind, are likely to be experienced as an impingement upon their therapeutic space.

In addition to client preferences, we therapists have preferences. There are clients with whom we may feel more or less comfortable disclosing, emotionally or factually. Since clients are not bound by confidentiality, anything we share (or any tears we shed) may be discussed with others. We must consider that whatever we share with our clients, through our words or our emotional expressions, could be repeated and that the client talking about us will do so from his or her perspective. Thus, a client who may be surprised by or uncomfortable with a therapist's teary eye may even describe the therapist as having "lost it," "broken down," or been a "crying mess" because that description is in keeping with the client's emotional reaction, even if it is disparate from our experience. (The best way to deal with this is to check in with clients, especially those you know less well, about the impact of any disclosures, perhaps especially emotional or unintentional ones.) In this way, we must trust our clients in order to feel comfortable with more vulnerable types of self-disclosure, such as crying or sharing something that is personal. In some cases, even if a client prefers more transparency, it may feel more of a risk than the therapist is willing to take. This may be especially true in certain practice settings, such as in small towns, college campuses, or when working with individuals with specific diagnoses who may otherwise have access to or know each other.

Lastly, what clients prefer and what is best for them can be incongruent. For example, a client may desire therapist self-disclosure as a way to avoid talking about him or herself. On the other hand, a client who dislikes any form of therapist self-disclosure may have difficulty dealing with other people's feelings in his or her personal relationships, too. Thus, many factors go into considering how best to use therapist self-disclosure: is this a client who will be put at ease by more transparency, or will such transparency feel like pressure to return caretaking in a way that feels burdensome to the client? Is this a client for whom some level of therapist self-disclosure may provide important corrective experiences within the therapeutic relationship in order to broaden such experiences to other relationships, or might therapist disclosure be a sort of complicit avoidance of the client's issues on the part of the therapist? Is this a client with whom the therapist feels comfortable disclosing? As we make educated guesses in each of our interventions, our best tool is always to talk about what happened and be open to shifting gears when we see that it is not leading to the progress we expect.

TEARS IN THERAPY: CASE EXAMPLES

Emily and My Eye-Opening Eye Infection

Emily had been struggling with feeling blocked in her therapy. She could not put her finger on it, but there were things she just could not talk about with me. For months we had been trying to pinpoint the issue, but it was my eye—tearing from infection, as described at the opening of this chapter—that sparked her insight.

"It feels uncomfortable to share really vulnerable things with you. I can talk easily with my friends because we're in the same boat: both people share. I feel like you would never let yourself cry here or show me what you feel because you're 'too ethical' and it makes me feel uncomfortable and less able to open up. I wish you would just cry if you felt like it," she said with a big sigh.

Emily was on to something here. To begin with, I'm not a big crier. But the previous year I had been going through an extremely hard time. My brother was a defendant in a criminal trial and I had missed quite a bit of work attending the trial. I was mentally and physically exhausted, living in a surreal state, and absolutely heartbroken by the situation. I felt emotionally raw, and was crying a lot in my free time. Nonetheless, I did my best to show up for my clients as the strong, present, and attentive therapist that I strived to be, not the crying one. Therapists should not cry about their own problems during their clients' therapy, nor appear emotionally fragile, right? I think that most of us would agree with this in theory. However, as I learned in my work with Emily, it is not necessarily always true.

Emily elaborated, "When you missed work because of your family emergency, I got that sense that I shouldn't ask you what it was, but I could tell it was something really bad. I could tell you weren't okay. That was really hard for me—I was worried about you. I was frustrated that I couldn't comfort you or be there for you. It felt unnatural and awful. And without knowing what you were going through, I made up horrible stories in my mind about what was going on."

Actually, I had put a lot of thought into what to share and what not to share—even consulting with colleagues about it—and concluded that shielding my clients from my raw emotions was the wisest choice. Thus I had decided to say the least amount I could get away with regarding my situation, explaining simply that I had to miss such-and-such sessions for a "family emergency." My clients kindly expressed their concern, but followed my cues to not ask too much.

When something happens in our personal lives that is truly emotionally taxing (e.g., a significant death, a health crisis), there is no roadmap for balancing our own needs with those of our clients. Every situation is unique. In this case, I worried that if I had talked about it while in the midst of feeling so vulnerable, I might have inappropriately poured out unfiltered emotions and thoughts. I did not want to take up my clients' time, overshare, or make anyone uncomfortable with the proverbial *too much information*. Also, I was not sure if I would have handled it well had clients reacted poorly to my disclosure; I would have needed to help them process their feelings about it and I was not in the state of mind to do so effectively. To avoid all of this, I defaulted to what I considered the most conservative choice: to disclose as little as was necessary.

By contrast, the therapist Emily had worked with in the past had cried freely in sessions; Emily said she could "read her like a book" and Emily appreciated this transparency. That therapist might have told her exactly what was going on, possibly cried about it, and then naturally moved on to what Emily needed to talk about. It seemed to work for them, but did not fit my style or comfort at that time. Yet Emily's response to my eye infection was causing me to reconsider. Emily and I had worked together for years now, and perhaps there were aspects of my style that, adhered to too rigidly, were hindering her progress in therapy. Perhaps she was right: in my efforts to be "ethical" and demonstrate "good boundaries," I had shared too little and caused her to feel shut out, leading to a disconnection and impasse in our work.

Therapy, by design, has a built-in imbalance with regard to self-disclosure: the client opens up, not the therapist; the relationship is designed to focus on the client's needs, not the therapist's. This is an essential and challenging paradigm for both sides. While our training teaches us to remove ourselves as much as possible in order to be objective, present, and focused for clients to give them the space to do their work, when we take that principle too literally or adhere to it too rigidly, we can lose the human element of therapy: the true caring, vulnerable, and mutual human connection that makes the process meaningful for client and therapist alike.

In this way, while it is not expected that therapists share information about their personal lives, not sharing enough can be interpreted as a way of demarcating a clear power differential in the relationship where the therapist gets to know about the client, yet the client does not get to know about the therapist, even when it is obvious that something is seriously wrong. That is hurtful to some clients. It may inadvertently replicate unhelpful family patterns in which the client felt invalidated or overly controlled by parents and other adults, or it could simply feel rejecting. My eye infection and Emily's response highlighted such a dynamic.

I contemplated all of this. Why wouldn't I be more open with Emily? Why had I not shared a little more? Having felt too vulnerable at the time, I overcompensated by not sharing enough. I could see now that it had affected our relationship in ways I had not anticipated. After exploring Emily's sense of being shut out by my non-disclosure, I made the decision to share with Emily what my family emergency had been. We then discussed why I had not felt able to talk about it at the time and also how I felt touched that she cared. I told her I was sorry she had felt so shut out and that she had had to manage her worries about me without my help. As I shared this, visceral emotion arose within me. I was not crying per se, but there was a noticeable difference in my voice. Emily could see this was a big step for me, and I could tell she felt honored that I was talking about it with her. In turn, this seemed to embolden her to open up about issues she had never talked about with anyone before. In the weeks to come, our work deepened; we were finally talking about aspects of Emily's life that were vital to our work but that had previously felt too risky, too vulnerable, for Emily to share.

Like all relationships, therapy relationships have ruptures and repairs. While less self-disclosure is a more cautious strategy, perhaps less likely to lead to an overt rupture, it can also be a lost opportunity and an impediment to progress. In Emily's case, my ultimate self-disclosure was the best way to repair and move through the rupture. Once she had articulated her frustration about my lack of disclosure, had I solely focused on her feelings about my non-disclosure, this might have perpetuated the distance Emily felt between us. Alternatively, had I shared about my family emergency while it was happening in the first place—likely with some tears, given the raw nature for me—it probably would have been well received by Emily, even helpful. Though I had chosen not to do so initially, we still had the opportunity for repair at a later date.

Tears and Mutuality: Breaking Through Trust Issues

Katie,[2] a college girl who was pushed into therapy by family and friends due to her eating-disorder symptoms, was guarded and ambivalent about change: she knew that how she was living was not working, but she could not imagine letting it go. She had seen me for months but the therapy felt stagnant, with her opening up in only limited and superficial ways. She admitted to having "trust issues" and expressed concern that a therapist would try to make her something that she was not, just as her parents had tried to do. To make matters worse, a prior therapist had broken confidentiality by reporting Katie's eating-disorder symptoms to her parents. Because of this, she was extremely reluctant to open up, even though a part of her did want the help. As we problem-solved about what might help her feel more comfortable, she suggested that knowing something about me might help her relax. I thought this over and explained that I did not mind self-disclosing to an extent, but I did not want conversations about me to be a way of avoiding talking about her. As long as I felt it was helpful, I told her, I was willing to find a way to co-create a therapeutic dynamic.

She began to ask me questions about myself: my own life lessons, my values, my journey into becoming a therapist, and when I responded comfortably and naturally she was both pleasantly surprised and put at ease. It seemed that my sharing helped her to relax, just as she had hoped it would, as well as sparked her own self-reflection, and she began to talk more openly. An unexpected consequence of the choice to foster this open dynamic between us was that my demonstration of comfort with myself provided a model of exactly what had been missing for Katie. She felt that while growing up it was unacceptable to simply be herself. She became what others wanted—upbeat, industrious, and always ready to help others—and used symptoms like restrictive eating or binge–purge cycles to control the expression of her true feelings. Her symptoms were self-validating: the harmful actions were reflective of what she felt she deserved, and were both comforting and self-punishing at the same time. This secret cycle of self-destructive behavior was uniquely hers, hidden behind the false self she presented to the rest of the world. In that sense, her eating disorder accomplished so much for her; the choice to give it up was not easy.

After months of resisting immersing herself in therapy, she announced she had a surprise for me and showed me a YouTube video. It involved people being prompted to talk about the person who was most influential in their lives, and then making a surprise telephone call to that person, telling the person what they meant to them. After watching the video together, Katie followed suit: she had written a beautiful passage for me, and read it aloud, telling me just what I meant to her and how my sharing, and my flexibility in working with her in the way she needed, had been profound for her. She was beginning to let me help her change. This was monumental.

As she read, my heart fluttered in my chest and I felt my eyes begin to fill with tears. I felt moved as she shared vulnerably from her heart, extending herself far beyond her comfort zone. This was unprecedented and completely unexpected. I was honored to be the first to witness this new level of emotional risk. I felt a sense of awe at how our slow but steady work toward building an open relationship had manifested in this magnificent way and I wanted her to know just how much this mattered to me. My tears were ready to pop.

What was I to do? Should I hold them back or let them go? Here, I was making a choice about emotional self-disclosure: I wanted to disclose to Katie the impact she had on me, too, and to give her the message that when she takes a risk—when she allows herself to be emotionally vulnerable and gives voice to her authentic self—there is an emotional reward: others are moved and intimacy deepens. I wanted to meet Katie where she was, to be there with her, with my feelings showing, and I believed that doing so was in line with our therapy goals, especially in increasing the trust and openness between us. As Katie looked up, she saw tears running down my face and I told her how touched I was by her beautiful words.

We looked back upon that day as pivotal in solidifying our relationship. It represented a new level of Katie trusting herself and our relationship, which helped her access the courage to do the work of transformation. In knowing I could be there as a real person, witnessing and supporting her, she felt safe enough to take the risk of making important changes.

Later in therapy, Katie reflected on the meaning of my tears that day and gave me permission to share her words here:

> *To me, a visceral emotional reaction is the ultimate truth. Non-verbal communication is so much more powerful because it's unable to be filtered like a statement. I've lived through years of saying I was fine when I was quite the opposite; had anyone only looked into my eyes, they would have recognized how much pain I was in. When you cried*

> *in response to my thoughts, this was the moment that I realized that our relationship wasn't just a job to you. In that moment, I recognized that you cared about me enough to allow yourself to be vulnerable and to display that level of emotion. Tears communicate emotion. You could have chosen to hold back your tears as much as possible, but instead you allowed them to fall free. You wanted me to see how much my words meant to you, in a vulnerable and emotional way. You wanted me to see how much I meant to you. You wanted me to see your truth. In therapy, showing that level of emotion is usually reserved for the patient. But that experience showed me a level of mutuality that I didn't think was possible in therapy. I needed to see that emotional self-disclosure is possible from a therapist in order to feel comfortable disclosing my true underlying emotions. That night I was converted from a skeptic to a believer in the benefit of therapy, pending you find the right match. I did.*

In reflecting on why I cried with Katie, it strikes me that one of the most moving aspects of therapy for me—indeed, the reason I am in this field—is to be a part of a person's transformation from symptomatic to healthy. As a fellow traveler, I know the courage and work it takes to change and grow. Being a therapist is an intimate and powerful experience that adds meaning to my own life. At moments when I witness my clients' epiphanies and find myself a part of their almost-magical change processes, I am always moved; sometimes I am moved to tears. In Katie's case, letting her see her impact on me made the moment even more transformational and memorable for us both.

CONCLUSION AND RECOMMENDATIONS

The most challenging aspects of therapy are not scripted: they arise organically from the relationship between the therapist and client. In *The Gift of Therapy*, Irvin Yalom includes a chapter entitled "Create a New Therapy for Each Patient" (Yalom, 2002). He writes of the importance of spontaneity in therapy, arguing that we need to both rely on our experience and therapeutic principles as well as tailor them to what is happening in the here and now with our clients. We use creativity in responding to our clients and meeting them where they are, and sometimes that includes sharing our emotions with our clients, including our tears.

Therapists behaving in a genuine manner—including allowing themselves to cry with, or in response to, their clients—can be potentially transformative for our clients and meaningful for us. If we view this within the framework of a self-disclosure decision, we can carefully assess how well self-disclosure fits into a particular therapy relationship in order to make an educated guess about how a client will react to our tears. Factors such as the client's preference for disclosure, the potential benefit of emotional disclosure for the client (which may or may not be congruent with the client's preference) and the therapist's comfort with emotional disclosure with this particular client are all important to consider.

As therapists, we are always making educated guesses about how to respond and intervene in a given moment. Of course, we are not always going to get it right. In addition, sometimes tears will be unintentional, emerging before we can make a decision to hold them back or not. If we make it a practice to talk about what our responses and interventions mean to our clients—particularly those as personal and potentially impactful as a therapist's tears—as well as consult our own reactions, we will likely be able to determine if this was a beneficial therapeutic choice or not. Even if it was not, therapy can move forward successfully with the ability to reattune, be curious and flexible, and make different choices in the future. In this way, when therapists' tears occur—whether they represent a rupture or an attuned response—both therapist and client will have learned something important.

NOTES

1. Name and all identifying case details have been changed to maintain anonymity and disguise the client.
2. While Katie (pseudonym) gave me permission to write about her case, all identifying information has been changed and significant case details altered to maintain her anonymity.

REFERENCES

Aron, L. (1996). *A meeting of minds: Mutuality in psychoanalysis*. Hillsdale, NJ: The Analytic Press.

Baldwin, M. (Ed.). (2000). *The use of self in therapy* (2nd ed.). New York, NY: The Haworth Press.

Bloomgarden, A., & Mennuti, R. (Eds.). (2009). *Psychotherapist revealed: Therapists speak about self-disclosure in psychotherapy*. New York, NY: Routledge Press.

Brown, L. (1994). *Subversive dialogues*. New York, NY: Basic Books.

Farber, B. (2006). *Self-disclosure in psychotherapy*. New York, NY: Guilford Press.

Hill, C. E., & Knox, S. (2002). Self-disclosure. In J. C. Norcross (Ed.), *Psychotherapy relationships that work* (pp. 255–266). New York, NY: Oxford University Press.

Knox, S., Hess, S. A., Peterson, D. A., & Hill, C. E. (1997). A qualitative analysis of client perceptions of the effects of helpful therapist self-disclosure in long term therapy. *Journal of Counseling Psychology, 44*, 274–283.

Kramer, C. H. (2000). Revealing ourselves. In M. Baldwin (Ed.), *The use of self in therapy* (2nd ed., pp. 61–96). New York, NY: The Haworth Press.

Linehan, M. (1993). *Cognitive-behavioral treatment of borderline personality disorder*. New York, NY: Guilford Press.

Maroda, K. J. (2004). *The power of countertransference* (2nd ed.). Hillsdale, NJ: The Analytic Press.

Miller, J. B., & Stiver, I. P. (1997). *The healing connection*. Boston, MA: Beacon Press.

Norcross, J. C. (2002). Empirically supported therapy relationships. In J. C. Norcross (Ed.), *Psychotherapy relationships that work* (pp. 3–16). New York, NY: Oxford University Press.

Rogers, C. (1989). The therapeutic relationship. In H. Kirschenbaum (Ed.), *The Carl Rogers reader*. New York, NY: Houghton Mifflin.

Shapiro, F. (1995) *Eye-movement desensitization and reprocessing*. New York, NY: Guilford Press.

Stricker, G., & Fisher, M. (Eds.). (1990). *Self-disclosure in the therapeutic relationship*. New York, NY: Plenum Press.

Treadway, D. (2009). For your client's sake: Practicing clinically constructive self-disclosure. In A. Bloomgarden & R. Mennuti (Eds.), *Psychotherapist revealed* (pp. 275–280). New York, NY: Routledge.

Wachtel, P. L. (2008). *Relational theory and the practice of psychotherapy*. New York, NY: Guilford Press.

Walker, M. (2004). How relationships heal. In M. Walker & W. Rosen (Eds.), *How connections heal* (pp. 3–21). New York, NY: Guilford Press.

Yalom, I. D. (2002). *The gift of therapy: An open letter to a new generation of therapists and their patients*. New York, NY: HarperCollins.

Zur, O. (2007a). *Boundaries in psychotherapy: Ethical and clinical explorations*. Washington, DC: American Psychological Association.

Zur, O. (2007b). The ethical eye: Don't let "risk management" undermine your professional approach. *Psychotherapy Networker, July/August*, 48–56.

Zur, O. (2009). Therapist self-disclosure: Standard of care, ethical considerations and therapeutic context. In A. Bloomgarden & R. Mennuti (Eds.), *Psychotherapist revealed* (pp. 31–51). New York, NY: Routledge.

Zur, O., Williams, M. H., Lehavot, K., & Knapp, S. (2009). Psychotherapist self-disclosure and transparency in internet age. *Professional Psychology: Research and Practice, 40*, 22–30.

CHAPTER 5

THERAPEUTIC IMMEDIACY: IF YOUR TEARS COULD SPEAK, WHAT WOULD THEY SAY?[1]

Mark J. Hilsenroth, Jason Mayotte-Blum, Klara Kuutmann, and Kristen L. Capps Umphlet

---

It was Ann's second-to-last therapy session. We had been working together for four years and the sessions had often been powerful and deep, with a focus on the here-and-now processing of emotion in the room. Now, after years of this work, I listened as Ann pondered our termination—one we jointly planned—this time by discussing the role of goodbye gifts. It struck me, in that moment, that she already had given me a gift, and I ventured to express as much to her—to express my gratitude for her gift of sharing herself so daringly, and to point out the gift she had given herself by making this time for herself.

"Don't make me upset!" Ann said, her eyes filling with tears as she listened to me express my appreciation.

"It's very emotional," I said. "And I'm not going to run from that." As I said that, tears came to my own eyes. This had been a theme in our work all along:

(continued)

> *(continued)*
>
> *therapy and our relationship had provided Ann a place to feel and express emotions that she felt her family and others avoided or scorned. Her first reaction was to run from the emotion, but, as I had tried to do throughout our work, I pressed on, staying with the feeling in the room, attempting to give her a place to try out ways of relating that were different from the emotionally avoidant family system she grew up in. This time, that meant the chance to say goodbye and grieve the loss of our relationship, as opposed to avoiding the painful feelings associated with endings, as she had done in relationships previously. I was moved myself by the poignancy of such feelings, both a sense of awe and respect for her investment and growth during this process as well as my own sadness regarding our goodbye.*
>
> *After a pause, Ann quietly agreed. "It is {very emotional}," she said, staying with the feeling, too, and crying herself. After a time, Ann explained of her tears, "They are just joining your tears."*

It is this type of comment—a here-and-now processing of the emotions happening in the therapy room between us—and the deeper discussions that accompany such comments on which this chapter will focus. More specifically, we will discuss how therapeutic immediacy can be utilized to both deepen the therapeutic process as well as make meaning of emotional transactions, such as tears, in therapy.

UNDERSTANDING THERAPEUTIC IMMEDIACY

As the therapeutic relationship is often experienced as an intimate, emotionally charged, asymmetrical, and nurturant relationship, psychotherapy is likely to activate many attachment-related patterns of thought, feeling, and conflict (Fonagy et al., 1996; Seligman & Csikszentmihalyi, 2000). Instead of viewing the treatment situation as primarily an interpretive stimulus field to be deconstructed, the therapeutic relationship can be understood as offering an active arena in which in vivo examination of client–therapist relational experiences may provide insight into some of the client's familiar patterns in close interpersonal relationships. By extension, it presents a unique relational training ground to brainstorm and attempt new models of thinking and relating, which may generalize to lasting personal changes (e.g., Blatt, 1990; Safran & Muran, 2000b).

A focus on the therapeutic relationship has been established as an important aspect of psychotherapy treatment across a wide range of therapeutic orientations (Beck, 1995; Freud, 1912; Norcross, 2011). In part due to the various different conceptualizations of an in-session focus on the therapeutic relationship in research, training, and practice, Hill (2004) developed an experience-near term, *therapist immediacy*, defined as disclosures of how the therapist is feeling about the client, him- or herself in relation to the client, or about the therapy relationship. Subsequently, in order to capture the more interactive and dyadic nature of the therapeutic relationship, this definition has been broadened to also reflect any client-initiated disclosures of feelings about the therapist or the client–therapist relationship, and the revised term of *therapeutic immediacy* has been suggested (Kuutmann & Hilsenroth, 2012). Thus, therapeutic immediacy involves any discussion about the relationship between therapist and client that occurs in the here and now, as well as processing in the moment anything that occurs in the relationship.

Typical examples of therapeutic immediacy include: (1) exploring parallels of how interpersonal and affective themes covered in other relationships during a session might be expressed or occur in the therapeutic relationship; (2) expressing an immediate in-session affect or association regarding the therapeutic relationship or treatment process; (3) asking one member of the therapeutic relationship (client or therapist) to take the perspective (thoughts or feelings) of the other; (4) asking one or both parties to reflect on/process what is happening in the immediate therapeutic interaction or feeling in the room; (5) exploring emotional experiences in the relationship that might have been avoided or gone unrecognized; (6) addressing a rupture event; (7) recognizing adaptive changes in functioning that occur in relation to the therapeutic relationship or treatment process; (8) explicitly supporting, affirming, and validating engagement, involvement, or greater experiencing in the therapeutic relationship or treatment process; and (9) processing the termination of the therapeutic relationship.

Thus, therapeutic immediacy may help to provide more adaptive (i.e., corrective) relational experiences with the therapist for the client by a focus on here-and-now awareness. In sum, consistent with the work of Hess (2002), Hill (2004), Wachtel (1993, 2008), McCullough and colleagues (2003), Safran and Muran (2000a), as well as Wachtel (1993, 2008), we would suggest that perhaps the most curative aspect of "here-and-now" in-session processing of the therapeutic relationship, rather than links to archaic, symbolic, or genetic associations, is the opportunity for an examined "in vivo" emotional relational interaction that can provide a much-needed template for more adaptive attachment strategies and interpersonal functioning.

In general, I (MH) am rarely moved to tears in a session, perhaps once or twice during the course of a given treatment, and in many treatments not at all. However, I believe that when a therapist is genuinely, authentically, and deeply moved in such a manner it may be detrimental to uncharacteristically restrict, avoid, or hide such a response. In fact, when I do have tears in my eyes during a session, I make it a point not to wipe them, and when tears roll down my cheek, I also refrain from wiping these away until after we have processed the meaning of that event in the session. This exploration and explicit discussion of tears represents an example of therapeutic immediacy that is often quite intense, and typically offers a powerful moment in the therapeutic relationship that lends itself to the opportunity for adaptive change. That is, the client becomes more able to recognize strong affect in others and him- or herself, and through this discussion is better able to tolerate affect that was once overwhelming and dysregulating.

TEARS IN THERAPY

Ann[2] (a pseudonym) was a 25-year-old single White female enrolled in a master's of arts program for Social Work. She originally entered psychotherapy experiencing four acute stressors within the same month: the death of her grandmother with whom she had a "special bond," the end of a three-year relationship with a boyfriend she found to be emotionally unresponsive, problems in her graduate program with regard to consistency and quality of her work, and difficulties with her externship supervisor, whom she found to be hypercritical and attacking. The initial four events occurred, in that order, all within four weeks, early into her second semester of graduate school. She was transferred to me after 14 months of therapy with a graduate trainee who left for her clinical internship. She was then a client of mine for over four years.

Ann reported that her first treatment was very useful in helping her through these acute crises, developing better emotional tolerance, transitioning from graduate school, and obtaining her first job in the social work profession. She also made progress in understanding maladaptive patterns, including her avoidance of experiencing and expressing her emotions. Furthermore, she had begun to express more compassion and acceptance of herself and her abilities. One significant change came in the form of her belief that "it's okay for me to sit here" and that doing things for herself, such as therapy, was not selfish and did not represent taking resources from those in greater need. However, she desired to become even more effective in these areas of functioning, and thus requested transfer to a new therapist when given that opportunity. Although improved, Ann continued to experience family and significant others in her life as generally unsupportive, uncommunicative, and inhibited regarding the expression of emotion. As such, she often experienced stressful events that left her struggling to cope with her emotions within the context of her family, relationships, and work environments. At the outset of treatment with me, Ann was also struggling with restricting her affective expression in the moment, leading to ever-increasing tension and stress that would ultimately give rise to impulsive actions within the context of her relationships (such as angry outbursts), particularly when she was feeling sad or lonely.

I first met Ann over a decade ago. I was 35 years old, a licensed and board-certified clinical Ph.D. psychologist with, at that time, nine years of postdoctoral therapy experience, and specific postdoctoral training in short-term dynamic psychotherapy and psychoanalysis. I would describe my clinical orientation as "contemporary psychodynamic," "relational," "supportive," "affect-focused," and "integrative," with significant clinical influences, including Wachtel (1993, 2008), McCullough et al. (2003), Strupp and Binder (1984), and Luborsky (1984). More specifically, I emphasize the following principles in my clinical work, as well as in individual and group supervision, and graduate courses on technique: (1) be an ally to your client's desire for change and underline even small steps of adaptive progress; (2) understand defense and resistance as old coping strategies, once useful, now gone awry; (3) support painful affect and experiences first, explore second; (4) follow the affect, then help the client to experience (in body), express, and explore its meaning; (5) explore how interpersonal and affective themes covered during the session play out across different relationships, especially in the therapeutic relationship; (6) explore the client's experience of this in-session process; and (7) the interactive present is the most helpful venue for changing cyclical maladaptive patterns. That is, rather than a place to repeat prior behavior, the therapeutic relationship is an arena where more adaptive relating is first practiced and then can be explored. Therefore, it is vital that the therapist recognize the client's adaptive relational attempts in the therapeutic work, and explore them every bit as much as maladaptive patterns that may emerge in the therapeutic situation.

Prior to treatment with me, Ann consented to participate in psychotherapy process and outcome research. As part of this research, Ann completed outcome measures prior to her first session as well as at the one-year mark, the three-year mark, the end of treatment (four years), and at an 18-month follow-up session. In addition, all sessions from Ann's four-year psychodynamic therapy were videotaped, transcribed verbatim, and coded for both therapeutic immediacy and affective intensity by a qualitative coding group of four graduate students (see Mayotte-Blum et al., 2012, for additional details). Because of this, we have the opportunity to draw upon research regarding session relevance and meaningfulness to the larger treatment process in examining how a therapist might process his or her own tears in therapy, i.e., how a therapist might use therapeutic immediacy to make meaning of a therapist's tears. Indeed, in our study, the two times that I became tearful during the course of the therapy with Ann were both rated to be among the top four most meaningful immediacy transactions in the entire treatment. To follow are excerpts and analyses of these two most clinically relevant and meaningful events to provide actual examples of the use of therapeutic immediacy in regard to a clinician's tears.

The following segment at the end of the first year of treatment with Ann involves therapeutic immediacy in what may be described in theoretical terms as a corrective emotional experience (Alexander & French, 1946). Ann had just finished describing very intense (i.e., sobbing deeply throughout) relational episodes with her family from a recent period of crisis that she characterized as being significantly neglectful and painful. When Ann attempted to express her feelings to her family, she reported being not only largely ignored, but also being attacked by her mother. In the process of listening to her story, I was impressed by Ann's attempt at actions that we had previously explored in therapy. That is, she tried to express and meet her needs effectively, as well as engage her family in a more adaptive manner in an attempt to improve their relationships. What struck me most was her sense that she was trying to interact in a new, healthy way, yet she still found herself in the same maladaptive pattern with her family whom she described as emotionally unavailable, avoidant, and withdrawn. When Ann initiated a discussion of emotions and relationships within that family system, she was viciously attacked for it. During her description of this process, I was moved by her expression of intense frustration, disappointment, hopelessness, utter futility, and sadness (i.e., grief), and her repeated questioning of whether she would ever get her needs met by her family, or if her family system would be amenable to change. As I witnessed her struggle with the implications of this pain and despair—that her needs, desires, and crises did not matter to her family, and by extension that she did not matter—I noticed my eyes tearing up and a tear rolling down my cheek.

At first, Ann seemed to ignore my emotional reaction, and when I asked what it was like to see tears on my face, she responded "I don't know," but then she acknowledged that she was "trying to ignore it."

At this point, I attempted to deepen the emerging therapeutic immediacy in the session:

Therapist: *So, me tearing up about that as you were crying about it . . .*
Client: *It's comforting.*
T: *Comforting. In what way. . . ?*
C: *'Cause it's sad. It's just sad. There's no, there's no, I don't know . . . I guess because sadness is hard for me . . . sadness is so hard for me that I'm like, ok, somebody's sad with me. I'm not on my own going, "Oh my God" . . . I'm always sad by myself so that's something that I'm used to . . . I guess more different this time, so this is different. (pulls out Kleenex)*
T: *Well, thanks, I appreciate that . . .*
C: *I'm like, you're making me cry now (crying) . . . because . . . (said in a very soft tone) . . . you're sad with me . . .*
T: *What's sad about this . . .*
C: *No, it's just . . . being joined and not just sitting here like . . . I'm having conversations with my Mom, and I'm sitting there crying, and she looks at me like stone cold, and you see her eyes getting red, and I know I do it . . . and you know, it's just . . . (large gesture) let that fucking emotion out! (said very loudly) Teach me! Teach me!*
T: *So you feel like something's going on . . .*
C: *You know what, 'cause it doesn't make it seem like it's a weakness . . . I guess that's kind of what it is. 'Cause in my family, it's still such a weak thing to do. (Softly) Such a weak thing to do.*
T: *So when I sit here and cry with you . . .*
C: *It reassures me that it's ok. That's really important, though, that is. Because I struggle so much with not being able to do that . . .*
T: *I know, but look at where you are and what you've done.*
C: *A crying mess . . .*
T: *No, no, you're feeling in important ways . . . you really are.*

I believe my open exploration of my own emotional response in this interaction was a powerful therapeutic mechanism. Indeed, the research team that analyzed this immediacy segment felt that my acknowledgment and expression of my own emotional experience were the critical events that set the stage for Ann to further explore her own emotions and judgments about them. By focusing on the experience of emotion in the room, I assisted Ann in engaging with me in a manner that was different from the familiar pattern of avoidance of affect, intimacy, and vulnerability that she reported so often occurred in her family.

While it may have been emotionally easier for me to avoid an exploration of these intense emotions in the room, I would have been colluding with and perpetuating the existing cyclical maladaptive relational pattern from which she was trying to break free. Furthermore, had I instead focused on defense interpretation—i.e., her initial attempts to avoid my response and its impact on the therapeutic relationship—that would have been misguided and detrimental to optimally maximizing this opportunity for growth. That is, had I adopted a critical (i.e., attacking) stance on what she was doing "wrong" (i.e., ignoring/avoiding), rather than exploring her attempts at mastery and underlining her adaptive efforts to experience and express herself in a manner that sought to increase intimacy, trust, and connectedness, I also would have been perpetuating the pattern of attacking that Ann reported with both her family and in work (i.e., her supervisor). In response, Ann expressed gratitude for my willingness to "be sad with her," which contradicted her belief, learned in her family, that sadness is weakness and should be avoided. Instead, she was provided with the experience of a man openly expressing his own emotions and vulnerability, in addition to sitting with her emotional experience, which may have helped to create hope for different experiences with men going forward (in contrast to her experience of a range of emotionally unavailable men in her life). In fact, she seemed eager for a different type of emotional-relational experience to help "teach her" a more adaptive mode of relating. Similarly, this interaction was important in offering a reframing or alternative viewpoint of events, namely, her sadness as "feeling in important ways" as opposed to her being "a crying mess."

In the fourth year of treatment, after overlapping vacations led to a four-week hiatus in therapy, Ann broached the topic of termination. First, she spoke with a good deal of self-efficacy regarding how well she had handled several potentially problematic situations and interactions during our break. She then wondered aloud what it would be like to not be in therapy any longer: did she "need" it and how well would she do without it? I approached this discussion with encouragement, support, and exploration. After agreeing to think more about the possibility of termination over the course of the week, Ann arrived at her next session having made the decision that she would like to begin the termination process and "give it a try without therapy." At that time, Ann and I contracted for a two-and-a-half-month period to focus on the termination process and set the date for our final session. This immediacy segment near the end of her next-to-last session is an example of how processing the therapeutic relationship is an important part of the termination process. I became tearful during this session, and our exploration of this issue provides a nice comparison with the segment above that had occurred three years earlier.

It is of note that, while some of the same issues are discussed and explored, this excerpt also provides a window into the trajectory of her emotional changes during the course of our work together. In this segment, Ann had just finished relating several discussions she had with friends and coworkers who had also been in psychotherapy regarding getting their therapist a goodbye gift, and what to do in a crisis after the termination of the therapy.

T: *Is that a question you want to ask me?*
C: Well, no 'cause I'm just not that person, that's like, oh let me get gifts for somebody. And I don't think I need to because the gift would be hopefully, you know, the work that we've done . . .
T: *Well, I think you're asking two questions, so let me respond to them. First, I think you've given me a very wonderful gift that's honored me every day that you've come in here . . .*
C: Don't make me upset! (starts to tear up)
T: *Well, it's, it's very emotional . . . and I'm not going to run from that either (tearing up)*
C: No, it is.
T: *I think that you've given a wonderful gift to me, but as important, to yourself. And I think that's the most important gift you could ever give, what you've given in this process over the time we've known each other. It's been a gift to me . . . it's been an honor, and it's been a gift to you to yourself, to show yourself how worthwhile you are. As far as the future goes, I guess this is how I look at those things and that is, once I'm your therapist, I'm always your therapist . . .*
C: Mm-hmm. Mm-hmm. (crying)
T: *I want you to feel that the door's always open to you.*
C: That's good.
T: *Sometimes I work with people and I don't hear from them for forever, and sometimes something comes up in their life and they want to give me a call and they want to come in for a few sessions, or sometimes they want to come in for more, longer than a few sessions, but that's okay. The door is always open to you. I hope that all the hopefulness you have, it all comes back to you and things work out wonderfully, and that you'll remember us in a good way and that it'll be helpful to you . . . that's what I hope . . . but bad things can happen, and circumstances can happen, and I always want you to know that you can call me. I guess we don't know what's going to happen in the future, but I want you to know that I'll be here for you, as long as I'm here.*
C: This is what I anticipated with you. One, you didn't disappoint me, and two, I didn't think you were ever going to abandon me . . .
T: *How did you hear what I just said?*

C: *I guess that's what I expected from you . . . this has been a very emotional thing, a very emotional thing. I have done my random little cries here just even in the past couple weeks . . . and you know like, "Fuck, is this a good idea with Dr. Mark?" But you know, I'm not going to know until, I mean I'm going through this process, and I'm saying goodbye, and just even hearing you say that makes me feel good. It's like, you know, this is a chapter that doesn't have to be ongoing, but every chapter ties into the next, and I just didn't think you would abandon me. I guess hearing that . . . and I'm like, "Oh, ok good!" (with large exhale). At least I have somebody I can trust that if I, God forbid, ever needed it . . .*

T: *What's it like to see me tear up in here? You've seen me tear up in here before . . .*

C: *It's nice. It's like, "look at this emotional man" . . . I mean, I've seen you tear when I'm at my most saddest . . . I've seen you tear when I'm like "Oh God!" (motions like crying hard) . . . um . . . I mean they're sad happy tears. It's a lot of good work and a lot of . . . again . . . you're very, you have a fatherly . . . I wouldn't say that you're a fatherly figure, but just you've always had that, like I know you care. You've watched me . . . in a parent kind of way where you watch your kid struggle . . . and again, not that I think you see me as some kid, but like, you've watched a person struggle and grow and been a part of that process that's kind of like, "Huh!" (large exhale). And it's letting go for you. I'm not the only person who has to let go, I'm here every Tuesday cursing you out in one way . . . people tend to miss that. (smiles)*

T: *What are your tears saying right now?*

C: *Um, they're happy . . . they are just joining your tears. It's kinda like, goodbye, like sweet sadness . . . it's not sad, that's just it . . . not sad, what's the phrase that they use? Back in the day, like my Grandma . . . bittersweetness? Is that the word?*

T: *So what do you think next week's going to be like? What do you think next week's going to be like as far as when the session ends . . .*

C: *I don't know . . . I might be crying . . .*

T: *Maybe me too. We're both crying right now at the end of this session . . .*

C: *I know. But they're not like "wah-wah" tears. I'm expressing myself . . . they're "expressing myself" tears . . .*

T: *Me too . . .*

My expression of gratitude for her engagement in the treatment process, and the genuine affect accompanying it, led to a deepening of Ann's exploration of emotion. Previously, during the last two months, Ann had discussed her feelings about termination, but not with as much intensity. In addition, while she had discussed the subject of loss both in and out of the therapeutic relationship, these explorations were not as prolonged and in depth as they would become in these final two sessions during and after this interaction. This session marked an important point in this process, where Ann discussed the impact of the loss of our relationship and the poignant sadness that may be conceptualized as evidence of her capacity to grieve. Ann previously stated that her past relationships had ended without an opportunity to talk about the loss and the associated feelings. I tried to maintain a focus on the subject of termination and provide gentle redirection when she attempted to move away from the affect in the termination process. I believe that my choice to allow myself to feel the fullness of our ending and to express these feelings to Ann, the depth and authenticity of which were evidenced by my tears, gave Ann the sense that she was not grieving alone. Had I expressed the same sentiments without genuine affect, or purposefully withheld my tears as I spoke, it is possible that Ann may not have felt the emotional safety to delve into her own vulnerable emotional experience, a process she described as her tears "joining [my] tears." My tears also had the impact, at this point in our work, of allowing Ann to see me as a separate person with my own emotions and experiences, a person who, as Ann stated, "has to let go," too. At the end of a treatment, this can be an appropriate and even important development of perspective and independence within the therapeutic relationship. During the final session, Ann identified this specific interaction as being particularly significant and powerful for her and her feelings about moving forward after therapy.

A unique aspect of Ann's case is that, because she agreed to participate in research, we have data regarding the effectiveness of our work, both short- and long-term, and information about what Ann felt to be most beneficial in our work, specifically with regard to therapeutic immediacy. Outcome measures showed that Ann made clinically significant progress in our work, moving from two standard deviations above the norm at the start of treatment into the normative range of function in global symptomology and interpersonal problems by the end of our work. These positive changes continued beyond the conclusion of treatment when assessed at 18 months post treatment. In a post-treatment interview with an independent clinician, which was part of the research protocol, Ann stated that talking about the therapeutic relationship (immediacy) was a vital aspect of the treatment. She noted that because her issues were mostly in relationships, discussing the therapeutic relationship enabled her to evaluate other relationships more confidently and effectively.

Ann also specifically identified the expression of feelings as memorable in the treatment. She stated that she cried through several sessions, which allowed her to experience feelings she has previously avoided. We might wonder whether my acceptance of my own tears in therapy facilitated Ann's acceptance of her own emotional expression. Through our discussions of my tears, Ann may have been able to view crying in a new way, different from the intolerance of affect that characterized her relationships with her family. Allowing myself to cry with Ann helped provide an experience of crying that could be seen as comforting and authentic, rather than a weakness. Because Ann's goals in therapy were specifically tied to difficulties in experiencing and expressing emotions in interpersonal relationships, my tears with Ann may have been particularly helpful in her specific case: she experienced real emotional exchanges with another person and, throughout these interactions, not only felt accepted but experienced the increasing closeness and comfort that can come with emotional authenticity. This may have given Ann a sense of efficacy and hope for what she could accomplish in relationships in the future. Indeed, when contacted three years post treatment, Ann reported that she was enjoying professional success and advancement, was in an enduring two-year romantic relationship with a man to whom she was engaged to be married, and was expecting the birth of her first child within the next few months, all signs that our work produced stable changes in Ann's functioning well beyond the end of therapy.

CONCLUSION AND RECOMMENDATIONS

This case provides a cross-sectional view of how therapeutic immediacy may be used to work with difficult clinical issues in the here and now of the therapeutic relationship, and specifically how it may be used to process a clinician's own tears to make the experience a positive—versus potentially detrimental, or simply neutral—experience. What we have hoped to portray in this chapter is that discussing therapists' tearfulness when it occurs—i.e., therapeutic immediacy—can be an important mechanism of change in the therapy. In the first clinical example above, my tears emerged as Ann was grappling with her fears that nothing in her family relationships would change despite her best efforts. While there was of course no way to change Ann's family in that moment, there was a way to change how Ann related to her pain, to help her feel less alone, and to help her experience new ways of relating to others that may be more satisfying than what she experienced with her family. My tears expressed my willingness to allow Ann to feel and to feel with her, something her family refused to do. By discussing my tears and the implications for our relationship explicitly, I refused to collude with the avoidant stance Ann's family had taken regarding difficult emotions and discussion of relationships, the precise stance that left Ann feeling so alone and hopeless. My tears and our purposeful discussion around them were thus the mechanism of change that allowed Ann to experience a different way of relating than the one that, in that very moment, she was fearful that she would never escape.

The context that led to my tears in the second clinical example above was somewhat different. My tears in the first example came as I experienced Ann's hopelessness about the potential for change in her family and her sense that she did not matter to her family—her "saddest" moment in our work together, as she would later comment. In other words, the feelings that led to my tears were Ann's and my tears represented our empathic connection. My tears in the second example actually expressed my own emotions as well; my own sadness, gratitude, and hopefulness as our work came to an end. My willingness to express my own emotions and Ann's ability to tolerate such an interaction were signs of the interpersonal progress she had made in our work, and also an agent of change as this facilitated an honesty around our goodbye that Ann had not previously experienced in relationships. When a therapist's tears do occur at termination, using therapeutic immediacy (i.e., processing one's own tears with the client) may be a way to deepen the adaptive process around the expression of grief, loss, and saying goodbye. As identified in Hill (2004), termination is a time when discussing immediate feelings in the relationship is necessary to avoid any tendencies by either client or therapist to steer clear of difficult feelings, such as grief and loss. Indeed, because termination is a time when therapists are actually experiencing a loss as well, a therapist's tears may be more likely to come at this time.

Though discussing one's own affect in the moment with a client can be an incredibly positive experience, and a useful catalyst in promoting relational growth, it is prudent to be thoughtful in this process. As in the case of Ann, the therapist must first be comfortable with his or her own affect, such that it can be expressed and experienced with a sense of safety and security. In addition, the therapist must be able to reflect on these feelings with the client. Doing so necessitates awareness of one's own limitations, as well as topics, affect, or interpersonal situations that might be personally dysregulating. In this case example, I was aware of my tears, and made a conscious clinical choice to bring the client's attention to them knowing the role of affective expression in her past, as well as her desire for something different in her future. The use of therapeutic immediacy was a decision based on knowledge of Ann's individual capacity to engage in this level of affective exploration, and the intervention was consistent with the goals of the therapy (e.g., Ann's desire to become more comfortable with strong feelings, and to engage in emotionally fulfilling relationships). It is important to note that my affect was expressed, yet still adequately modulated, such that I was not relying on the client to emotionally care for me in the moment. Rather, I was in a position to share my feelings with her, providing us with the opportunity to further explore the meaning and nature of these affective issues within our relationship, and contrast that with previous cyclical patterns of relating. Sharing my tears helped her to experience affective insight both in relation to herself and others.

Combined with a supportive and attentive approach, the collaborative exploration of client–therapist relational experiences tills fertile ground for therapeutic insight and relational growth. Focusing on in-session affective and relational experiences that emerge in the client–therapist interaction, such as a client's or therapist's tears, can foster therapeutic depth, and aid in the development and maintenance of a collaborative, affectively engaged relationship that may serve as a template for new adaptive relational experiences in a client's life. Encouraging such relational exploration *in the moment* actively disrupts cyclical patterns or ways of coping that at one time may have been helpful, but now prevent the client from engaging in fulfilling, meaningful relationships. In sum, the effective use of therapeutic immediacy allows the client to gain experience in tolerating, experiencing, and expressing affect, as well as giving voice to what may have once been avoided or found to be overwhelming by the client. This process allows clients to practice the change they hope to effect in future relationships and with themselves.

NOTES

1. Portions of this chapter are drawn from an earlier publication of the authors: Mayotte-Blum, J., Slavin-Mulford, J., Lehmann, M., Pesale, F., Becker-Matero, N., & Hilsenroth, M. (2012). Therapeutic immediacy across long-term psychodynamic psychotherapy: An evidence-based case study. *Journal of Counseling Psychology, 59(1)*, 27–40.
2. Ann consented to use material from her treatment in a case-study format.

REFERENCES

Alexander, F., & French, T. M. (1946). The corrective emotional experience. *Psychoanalytic therapy: Principles and application.* New York, NY: Ronald Press.

Beck, J. S. (1995). *Cognitive therapy: Basics and beyond.* New York, NY: Guilford Press.

Blatt, S. J. (1990). Interpersonal relatedness and self-definition: Two personality configurations and their implications for psychopathology and psychotherapy. In J. L. Singer (Ed.), *Repression and dissociation: Implications for personality theory, psychopathology and health* (pp. 299–335). Chicago, IL: University of Chicago Press.

Fonagy, P., Leigh, T., Steele, M., Steele, H., Kennedy, R., Mattoon, G., . . . Gerber, A. (1996). The relation of attachment status, psychiatric classification, and response to psychotherapy. *Journal of Consulting and Clinical Psychology, 64*(1), 22–31.

Freud, S. (1912). The dynamics of transference. In J. Strachey (Ed. & Trans.), *The standard edition of the complete psychological works of Sigmund Freud Volume XII* (1911–1913): The case of Schreber, papers on techniques and other works (pp. 97–108). London, UK: Hogarth Press.

Hess, J. A. (2002). Distance regulation in personal relationships: The development of a conceptual model and a test of representational validity. *Journal of Social and Personal Relationships, 19*, 663–683.

Hill, C. E. (2004). *Helping skills: Facilitating exploration, insight, and action* (2nd ed.). Washington, DC: American Psychological Association.

Kuutmann, K., & Hilsenroth, M. J. (2012). Exploring in-session focus on the patient–therapist relationship: Patient characteristics, process and outcome. *Clinical Psychology and Psychotherapy, 19*(3), 187–202.

Luborsky, L. (1984). *Principles of psychoanalytic psychotherapy: A manual for supportive expressive treatment.* New York, NY: Basic Books.

Mayotte-Blum, J., Slavin-Mulford, J., Lehmann, M., Pesale, F., Becker-Matero, N., & Hilsenroth, M. (2012). Therapeutic immediacy across long-term psychodynamic psychotherapy: An evidence-based case study. *Journal of Counseling Psychology, 59*(1), 27–40.

McCullough, L., Kuhn, N., Andrews, S., Kaplan, A., Wolf, J., & Hurley, C. (2003). *Treating affect phobia: A manual for short-term dynamic psychotherapy.* New York, NY: Guilford Press.

Norcross, J. C. (2011). *Psychotherapy relationships that work: Evidence-based responsiveness* (2nd ed.). New York, NY: Oxford University Press.

Safran, J. D., & Muran, J. C. (2000a). *Negotiating the therapeutic alliance: A relational guide.* New York, NY: Guilford Press.

Safran, J. D., & Muran, J. C. (2000b). Resolving therapeutic alliance ruptures: Diversity and integration. *Journal of Clinical Psychology, 56*(2), 233–243.

Seligman, M. E. P., & Csikszentmihalyi, M. (2000). Positive psychology: An introduction. *American Psychologist, 55*(1), 5–14.

Strupp, H. H., & Binder, J. L. (1984). *Psychotherapy in a new key: A guide to time-limited dynamic psychotherapy.* New York, NY: Basic Books.

Wachtel, P. L. (1993). *Therapeutic communication: Principles and effective practice.* New York, NY: Guilford Press.

Wachtel, P. L. (2008). *Relational theory and the practice of psychotherapy.* New York, NY: Guilford Press.

CHAPTER 6

THE PSYCHOANALYST'S TEARS: FROM ABSTINENCE TO AUTHENTICITY

Patricia Harney

My relationship with psychoanalysis started formally when I was a college student. I worked for a professor, a psychoanalyst, who consulted to a halfway house for adults with psychiatric illness. This was in the 1980s, when psychoanalytically oriented treatments were still prominent in community mental health. The analyst ran therapy groups for the halfway-house residents, adults with schizophrenia, serious bipolar disorder, severe autism and so on. Students like me sat in as participant-observers. In my first experience of this group, Dr. M asked residents and students to share our thoughts about or experiences with therapy. When my turn came to speak, I became anxious. I mentioned these feelings and went on to say that I was always curious about whether therapy would be useful for me. As I said this, I began to cry. Internally mortified but outwardly calm, I thought to myself, "Well, now I have proven that I need therapy!"

This professor became an important mentor to me and guided me along the way to graduate school. I lived in fear, however, that he would describe me as "emotionally labile" on letters of reference because of my tears, that he would see me as unfit to become a psychoanalyst. As I prepared to graduate from college and begin my doctoral studies, he told me that he knew from that first meeting—the one in which I cried—that I would make a very good psychologist.

I begin with this recollection because it contains strains of the conflicting notions held by psychoanalytic theory and psychoanalysts regarding crying in the consulting room. Even as a college student, I held implicit principles of abstinence and neutrality as rules that guided treatment. Just as I graduated from college, however, the late 1980s saw a significant turn in psychoanalytic thinking. In this chapter, I will review past and contemporary psychoanalytic concepts as they pertain to the psychoanalyst's tears. A review of original concepts contextualizes the stigma associated with the therapist's tears. Contemporary concepts help us consider the ways in which the therapist's tears can catalyze or derail therapeutic action. A clinical example from my own practice will be used to illustrate contrasting ways to understand the emergence of the therapist's tears and their impact on the treatment process.

PSYCHOANALYTIC THEORY AND TEARS

On Freud, Abstinence, and Neutrality

In his paper on the technique of psychoanalysis, Freud (1913) outlined specific principles by which the analyst should guide his or her attitude and behavior. He considered the concept of abstinence as central to the efficacy of treatment. Abstinence refers to the belief that the therapist should avoid attitudes or interactions that gratify the client's emotional needs. Gratification would foreclose the opportunity to explore those needs and the client's defenses against them. A treatment relationship that is less emotionally comfortable allows the client's needs, wishes, and fears to rise to the surface. The therapist restrains his or her emotional freedom to create space for the client's emotional freedom to expand.

In this classical psychoanalytic view, the therapist guards the therapeutic space to allow the client's transference—his or her fantasies, wishes, and fears about the therapist—to unfold. Different branches of psychoanalytic theory developed over the course of the 20th century, from ego psychology (e.g., A. Freud, 1937), to object relations (e.g., Klein, 1937) to self psychology (Kohut, 1977), yielding different models of the unconscious mind and different views of therapeutic action. Yet, the view of the treatment situation as one in which the therapist maintains or at least strives toward emotional neutrality remained unchanged. Countertransference—the full range of the therapist's feelings, attitudes, and fantasies toward the client—was regarded as an obstacle to the treatment, a result of the therapist's unresolved conflicts or fantasies (Gabbard, 1990; Lemma, 2003; Mitchell, 1997, 2000). A therapist's inability to mask or contain feelings would render him or her ill-suited to the analytic task. In fact, several authors have noted the irony that, while Freud identified transference very early in his theorizing as a vital concept and tool in treatment, its corollary, countertransference, was virtually ignored as a useful tool until the 1950s (Racker, 1957; Sandler, 1976).

This critical change in the view of countertransference emerged in the 1950s, when Paula Heinmann (cited in Sandler, 1976) theorized that the analyst's feelings may be a useful clue in understanding the client's inner world. Through the mechanism of projective identification, a client unconsciously exerts subtle pressure on the analyst to feel and perhaps act in certain ways that have particular meaning to the client. Heinmann argued that the therapist must *sustain*, not *rid*, him- or herself of such feelings, in order to more deeply understand the client's inner experience; these feelings often represent repetitions from formative relationships early in the client's life. Taking this concept further, Sandler (1976) argued that the analyst should maintain "free-floating responsiveness"; that is, an internal attitude of acceptance of all the feelings that arise in her- or himself. Sandler clearly stated that unexpected feelings on the analyst's part were not necessarily a result of the analyst's limitations of competence but rather an acceptance of the response that the client evokes in her or him.

The Interpersonal and Relational Traditions and the Concept of Enactment

What role does the analyst's personhood, or subjectivity, have in treatment efficacy? Since the late 1970s and early 1980s, this question has been asked and answered in a variety of ways in the psychoanalytic literature. Gill (1983) explored the distinctions between theoretical frames and technical stances in his essay on "The Interpersonal Paradigm and the Degree of the Therapist's Involvement," noting that classical Freudians *tend toward* minimizing the role of the analyst's participation, and interpersonalists (and perhaps those analysts who later came to refer to themselves as relational) *tend toward* a fuller participation. He noted, however, that theoretical paradigm and therapist stance do not always line up in this manner. Hoffman (1998) described a stance in which the analyst "has an ongoing sense of the embeddedness of his or her actions in a relational field in which transference and countertransference continually shape and partially illuminate each other" (p. 182). From his perspective, the therapist's ability and willingness to be open, honestly expressive, and disclosing were important—even essential—aspects of relational psychoanalysis.

Stephen Mitchell (1988, 1997, 2000) wrote extensively on the relational turn in psychoanalysis and dismantled the view of abstinence as a sacred principle. A key tenet in Mitchell's view of therapeutic action is *affective permeability*: the necessity of affective exchanges that are alive, deep, and resonant between both participants in the therapeutic dyad. The therapist's openness to the boundaryless, affective experience allows for a kind of emotional contagion that can assist the analyst in understanding the deepest, and often dissociated, aspects of the client's experiences (Mitchell, 2000). He argued, "Unless the analyst affectively enters the client's relational matrix or, rather, discovers himself within it . . . the treatment is never fully engaged, and a certain depth within the analytic experience is lost" (p. 293). Accordingly, a generation of writers have discussed the importance of the therapist's openness to authentic, emotionally alive exchanges between therapist and client (Davies, 1994; Ehrenberg, 1992; Maroda, 1991).

With a theoretical shift toward an understanding of the therapist's active, emotional engagement, the concept of enactment has risen to critical importance over the last two decades. Enactment is typically understood as the behavioral expression of the therapist's countertransference feelings. More specifically, enactments are considered to be the "therapist's inadvertent actualization of the patient's fears and fantasies" (Ivey, 2008, p. 24). Some see enactments as the client's unconscious attempt to recruit the therapist to feel and respond in certain ways that are consistent with his or her hopes or fears. In this sense, enactments are the therapist's verbal and non-verbal unintentional reactions to the client's transferences. Whether enactments represent a growth opportunity or an obstacle for the treatment is a matter of debate, with relational theorists tending to hold the former view and classical or Kleinian theorists tending to hold the latter (Ivey, 2008). Ivey (2008) provides a comprehensive summary of the concept of enactment, as well as a review of current controversies surrounding it.

In some respects, it is easy to see how the therapist's tears may be considered a countertransference enactment. Even if today's clients do not expect therapists to maintain a "blank slate" demeanor, they do expect a certain amount of emotional equilibrium from their therapists. The therapist's tears are the behavioral expression of feelings that the therapist cannot contain. Any unexpected expression of affect might give rise to transferential fantasies, such as "Am I too much to bear?" "Can she really handle me?" "I must be special for her to be this open with me." Regardless of the client's fantasy, the therapist's tears surely signal the therapist's vulnerability. And the therapist's vulnerability has assumed a more important role as traditional analytic authority has been deconstructed (Mitchell, 1997, 2000).

In his review, Ivey (2008) considers debates between classical, Kleinian, and relational theorists about enactments, in particular whether enactments are a necessary part of the treatment process or a hindrance to the work.

With respect to tears, therefore, classical and Kleinian theorists may be likely to see the therapist's tears as a break in the analytic attitude which disturbs the analyst's ability to think about the client. Such breaks in attitude intrude upon the opportunity for clients to identify their own thoughts, feelings, and beliefs. From this perspective, the emergence of the therapist's tears is the therapist's defensive maneuver away from the client's pain. Alternatively, from a relational perspective, the therapist's tears can represent an authentic, spontaneous engagement that allows clients to reclaim feelings and associated memories or fantasies that they disown or dissociate. Ivey (2008) argues persuasively that enactments may represent either an opportunity or a hindrance. Accordingly, the therapist's tears may be seen in this light.

Interpersonal theorist Philip Bromberg's (1996) view of the self offers a broad scaffolding from which to consider the meanings and mechanisms of enactments. Bromberg's understanding of self is based foundationally on the notion of multiplicity. He argues, "self-experience originates in relatively unlinked self-states . . . the experience of being a unitary self is an acquired, developmentally adaptive illusion" (Bromberg, 1996, p. 512). He further contends that normal personality structure is shaped by the processes of dissociation as well as by repression and intrapsychic conflict. A personal sense of authenticity depends upon the negotiation of tension between one's distinct self-states and the system as a whole. Moreover, in his view, dissociation allows for a person to function well "when full immersion in a single reality, a single strong affect, is called for or wished for" (Bromberg, 1996, p. 512).

Dissociation is also an interpersonal process, and can exist dynamically between client and therapist. Aspects of the client's dissociated experience are often enacted with the therapist and serve as an important avenue of communication. In order to decode such communications, Bromberg recommends that the therapist track his or her subjective experience of the therapeutic relationship and its ever-shifting qualities. At best, the therapist will monitor his/her awareness of shifting self-states in the client and in the therapist, and then carefully consider whether and how to communicate this awareness to the client. However carefully the therapist tracks the ever-shifting context of multiple self-states between both people, surprises abound—in sudden shifts of affect, association, memory, and self–other representation.

CRYING IN THE CONSULTING ROOM

While the psychoanalytic literature has expanded on the concept of countertransference in the way described above, very little is actually written directly about the analyst's tears. In fact, little more is written about the client's tears (Alexander, 2003). Clinical vignettes in contemporary analytic writing illustrate all manners of sudden shifts in affect and association on the part of the analyst, toward exploration of configurations of analytic engagement that contrast starkly with classical models. Many examples are dramatic and frequently referenced: Davies' (1994) essay, "Love in the Afternoon," in which the analyst declares her attraction to her client; Ehrenberg's (1992) expression of anger toward her client during a time of Ehrenberg's mourning; Hoffman's (2000) letters between himself and a client in the aftermath of Hoffman's triple-bypass surgery. There are equally instructive anecdotes of a less dramatic nature—see, for instance, Slochower's (2003) article on the quiet disengagements we make by temporarily and secretly withdrawing our attention away from clients.

Interestingly, however, I have been hard pressed to find vignettes in which the analyst cries. In those articles I have found in which therapists reference their own tears, the crying is alluded to without much ado. For example, Saakvitne (2002) refers to the many times she found herself welling up with clients in the aftermath of the September 11, 2001 terrorist attacks. More recently, in his beautiful meditation on his work with a dying analysand, Marguiles (2014) notes with a quiet dignity that he and his client often teared up together. Harry Guntrip (1986), in his account of being in analysis with Fairbairn, makes reference to Fairbairn's tears at the end of treatment when he writes,

> As I was finally leaving Fairbairn after the last session, I suddenly realized that in all the long period we had never once shaken hands, and he was letting me leave without that friendly gesture. I put out my hand and at once he took it, and I suddenly saw a few tears trickle down his face. *I saw the warm heart of this man with a fine mind and a shy nature.*
>
> (p. 454)

He says nothing more of his analyst's tears. And McWilliams (1994), in a discussion of the advantages of using the couch, writes that:

> [the couch] allows the therapist the freedom to respond internally to the client's material without self-consciousness: to fantasize, to respond affectively, even to weep without worrying that the client will be distracted from the internal processes by the therapist's emotional reactivity.
>
> (p. 242)

Her brief allusion to the analyst weeping certainly implies that tears can occur in treatment, but she says nothing more about such tears.

What could account for this relative silence on the topic of the therapist's tears in psychoanalytic writing? On the one hand, it seems that enactments involving the therapist's declarations of love, sexual attraction, and aggression are all less taboo in clinical discussion than those involving the therapist's tears. Alternatively, perhaps clinicians do not write much about the moments we cry with clients because they seem particularly sacred.

Historically, what analysts have theorized about the *client's* tears is not appealing. Tears have signified dependency, or symbolized urination and as such, a displacement of sexual conflicts (Greenacre, 1945; Lofgren, 1966). This history of characterization might make it difficult to bring such an analysis upon ourselves! In contemporary psychoanalytic theory, some might consider crying in the consulting room just another variation on the endless possibilities of enactment. I argue, however, that the therapist's act of shedding tears is a special case of enactment. Consider that tears are the only bodily secretion that we share publicly. The only time our clients actually see something from inside of our body come out is when we cry. We can easily feel shame when our faces stain with tears, as if we are naked before the eyes of the other. Crying is tinged with shame, culturally and developmentally. In writing this chapter, I am reminded of my own early experiences with tears and shame—for instance, the one "bad" grade I received on my kindergarten report card was in the category of self-control. The teacher wrote in the comment margin "cries too easily." Naturally, when I received that report card, I cried.

For these reasons, a therapist crying in the consulting room creates a special kind of intimacy unlike any other enactment (that is not an outright, physical boundary violation). The material fact of tears is unambiguous (even if clients "choose" not to notice them), and our willful control over their expression often does not exist. These features, the particular intimacy and our usual absence of control, are among the reasons it is vital for us to formulate ways of understanding and evaluating our crying on the treatment process.

"I Don't Want to Rain on Your Parade": A Clinical Vignette

Ms. R[1] was a woman I treated in psychotherapy for almost ten years. She had a history of multiple traumas, and presented with sequelae of complex posttraumatic stress. Our work together was arduous, owing to a deeply entrenched sense she had of herself as poisonous. Suicidal thoughts cast a constant shadow. At times, she would describe feeling the urge to cut herself in order to release the toxins she felt ran through her veins. The work for both of us was painful but ultimately gratifying, as she in time shifted toward a more consistently embodied self-compassion, and a slowly building sense of trust in others.

In our ninth year of work, she completed a program of graduate study that culminated in an excellent job offer in a far-away region of the country. And so our work together necessitated conclusion, as she had no plans to return to my locale. We knew of this impending move for several months, and in her deliberation about whether to accept the job and make this life change, she never once initiated a discussion of its import for our relationship and work together. I waited patiently for weeks as she discussed the pros and cons of the opportunity. She finally decided to accept, a choice that seemed quite reasonable, all things considered, and in fact quite brave. As she deliberated, however, I felt a growing swell of tension from the absence of any reference in her considerations to our relationship. I, in turn, deliberated about whether, when, and how to bring us into her conscious thought, as I hoped she would come to this on her own, and as I worried that she would experience an inquiry initiated by me about our relationship as a self-serving distraction from her growing sense of competence and autonomy.

Ultimately, I could wait no more. I ventured to say, "Have you thought about how it will be for you for us to say goodbye?" My eyes began to well. She looked shocked. "I thought we would just do phone sessions . . ." My tension peaked and I burst into tears as I said, "No. We can't." We often hear the phrase "projectile vomiting." I have never heard of "projectile tears," but that is what came out of me that day. Tears did not stream down my face; they shot directly to my client seated across from me. She, in turn, broke down crying. From there, we discussed both the logistical aspects of our need to say goodbye, and the wider dimensions of how this moment came to be—my tears and their possible meanings.

Classical, Kleinian, and relational psychoanalytic viewpoints illuminate different possible mechanisms, meanings, and consequences of my outburst. From a classical perspective, we might consider the role that my own unresolved conflicts regarding separation, loss, and abandonment contributed to my emotional expression. We also might consider the narcissistic difficulty that I had with my diminishing importance in Ms. R's life. I clearly broke the rules of abstinence and neutrality with the betrayal of my emotional response to my client. To the extent that the client was "testing" me by acting as if our relationship and work had no bearing on her decision to move, she may have aimed to see whether and to what extent she was important to me. My tears, then, may have gratified her wish to verify her importance to me. In this sense, my outburst may have foreclosed an opportunity to explore this wish and its corresponding fears.

A Kleinian analyst might regard Ms. R's avoidance of discussion of our relationship as an act of aggression that she could not own. She may have needed to make me disappear, symbolically kill me off, in order to feel that she could move on with her life. By crying, I cracked from the pressure of her disavowed aggression. Rather than containing her aggressive maneuver and securing myself as a steady maternal figure, my tears indicated vulnerability, perhaps weakness, in my ability to sustain her attack. This display of vulnerability might lead clients to dilute the intensity of their feelings for the therapist's sake, or for the sake of stabilizing the treatment situation.

When thinking about Ms. R's refusal to acknowledge our relationship from a relational perspective, we would consider what aspects of her experience she was dissociating, and what aspect of my unconscious life located was by what she could not own. In years past, Ms. R told me that she always felt rejected when a relationship ended, *even and sometimes especially* if she was the one ending it. Anticipation of the feeling of rejection often kept her from ending relationships. In this moment in treatment, then, she needed to protect herself from this feeling in order to follow her desire to leave, a desire that seemed in so many respects developmentally appropriate. But the feeling of rejection was not gone; instead, I was pressed into service as the container of this feeling.

The concept of projective identification is necessary but not sufficient in understanding the intensity of the feelings I ultimately expressed. In addition to the subtle interpersonal pressure that Ms. R exerted, my own life experiences created a readiness to respond in the way I did. In my teenage years, I had a beloved music teacher. For reasons related to time and money, she and I both had to fight hard to work together. Abruptly, this teacher was offered a job on another continent, and for her own intrapsychic reasons, she refused to say goodbye to me, but rather, kept alive a hope that she would do so, until that opportunity evaporated. Her refusal to say goodbye to me ushered in a period of depression, and a halt in my musical studies. While I certainly was not thinking of this experience in the moment with Ms. R, in my unconscious lived my direct experience with the inhibiting impact that a refusal to say goodbye could have. I believe that Ms. R's refusal to acknowledge our necessary goodbye, coupled with the intensity of our years of work together, created a specific activation of feeling within me that led to an outburst so unlike what I had experienced with any client previously. My tears, catalyzed by the tension I felt from the client's disavowal and activated by the specific unconscious experiences residing within me, jettisoned these feelings from my internal world back to the interpersonal field between us, where we could share the feelings about our necessary goodbye that seemed too much for either one of us to bear alone.

All three analytic perspectives outlined here offer value to an understanding of my tearful enactment. Emotional equilibrium *is* necessary on the therapist's part for many reasons, but above all, in order to maintain a consistent focus on the client's needs. Departures from that equilibrium should be examined carefully. A therapist's emotional expressions or outbursts can intrude on the space designed to explore the client's feelings, fears, and fantasies. Moreover, it is critical that we don't break or retaliate in response to a client's attacks, especially those attacks that are covert. The more covert an attack, the more the client is defended against the feelings underneath. However, with equilibrium as our baseline, it can be quite productive to explore departures from that baseline when enactments occur. A therapist's openness to their countertransference, not only their thoughts, feelings, and fantasies, but also their embodied countertransference (Stone, 2006), enables a deeper and more alive therapeutic dialogue.

While Ms. R and I spent little time explicitly discussing the impact of my crying, I aimed to observe whether her flow of associations or feelings transformed in any way after my tears. As in many aspects of clinical work, observable changes in affect, posture, or thought process offer clues to the client's experience as much as, if not more so than, their explicit verbalizations. Following my tears, Ms. R began to cry, and she was able to talk more fully about her feelings about our termination. It seemed that my own tears facilitated her expression of affect, both non-verbally (tears) and verbally. If her flow of thoughts or feelings slowed or halted, I would have been concerned about the possible inhibiting effect of my tearfulness.

CONCLUSION AND RECOMMENDATIONS

By their nature, enactments are spontaneous, unplanned, and can be explored only from the vantage point of "the rear view mirror" (Renik, 2006). We never plan to cry with our clients; it just happens sometimes. It may happen to some of us more than to others, owing to differences in our somatic receptivity (Stone, 2006). And so, with respect to the question, "Is crying an opportunity or a hindrance to the treatment?" I believe the question itself is not useful. We don't have a choice when we cry. The matter then becomes *how* we use it. That requires a commitment to exploring, in the privacy of our minds, the fullest range of our countertransference, careful attention to our somatic experience, and assiduous listening to and observing our clients' verbal and non-verbal responses.

NOTE

1. Details of Ms. R's case have been changed to maintain confidentiality.

REFERENCES

Alexander, T. (2003). Narcissism and the experience of crying. *British Journal of Psychotherapy, 20*(1), 27–38.

Bromberg, P. M. (1996). Standing in the spaces: The multiplicity of self and the psychoanalytic relationship. *Contemporary Psychoanalysis, 32,* 509–535.

Davies, J. M. (1994). Love in the afternoon: A relational reconsideration of desire and dread in the countertransference. *Psychoanalytic Dialogues, 4*(2), 153–170.

Ehrenberg, D. B. (1992). *The intimate edge: Extending the reach of psychoanalytic interaction.* New York, NY: W.W. Norton.

Freud, A. (1937/1992). *The ego and the mechanisms of defence.* London: Karnac Books.

Freud, S. (1913). On beginning the treatment: Further recommendations on the technique of psycho-analysis, I. *Standard edition, 12,* 121–144. London: Hogarth Press.

Gabbard, G. O. (1990/2014). *Psychodynamic psychiatry in clinical practice* (5th ed.). Washington, DC: American Psychiatric Publishing.

Gill, M. (1983). The interpersonal paradigm and the degree of the therapist's involvement. *Contemporary Psychoanalysis, 19*(2), 200–237.

Greenacre, P. (1945). Urination and weeping. *American Journal of Orthopsychiatry, 14,* 62–75.

Guntrip, H. (1986). My experience of analysis with Fairbairn and Winnicott. In P. Buckley (Ed.), *Essential papers on object relations* (pp. 447–468). New York, NY: New York University Press. (Original work published in 1975.)

Hoffman, I. (1998). *Ritual and spontaneity in the psychoanalytic process: A dialectical-constructivist view.* Hillsdale, NJ: The Analytic Press.

Hoffman, I. (2000). At death's door: Therapists and patients as agents. *Psychoanalytic Dialogues, 10*(6), 823–846.

Ivey, G. (2008). Enactment controversies: A critical review of current debates. *The International Journal of Psychoanalysis, 89*(1), 19–38.

Klein, M. (1937/2002). *Love, guilt, and reparation.* New York, NY: The Free Press.

Kohut, H. (1977). *The restoration of the self.* Chicago, IL: The University of Chicago Press.

Lemma, A. (2003). *Introduction to the practice of psychoanalytic psychotherapy.* Chichester, UK: John Wiley.

Lofgren, L. B. (1966). On weeping. *Journal of the American Psychoanalytic Association, 47*, 375–381.

Marguiles, A. (2014). After the storm: Living and dying in psychoanalysis. *Journal of the American Psychoanalytic Association, 62*, 863–905.

Maroda, K. (1991). *The power of countertransference: Innovations in analytic technique.* Chichester, UK: John Wiley.

McWilliams, N. (1994). *Psychoanalytic diagnosis.* New York, NY: Guilford Press.

Mitchell, S. A. (1988). *Relational concepts in psychoanalysis: An integration.* Cambridge, MA: Harvard University Press.

Mitchell, S. A. (1997). *Influence and autonomy in psychoanalysis.* Hillsdale, NJ: The Analytic Press.

Mitchell, S. A. (2000). *Relationality: From attachment to intersubjectivity.* Hillsdale, NJ: The Analytic Press.

Racker, H. (1957). The meanings and uses of countertransference. *Psychoanalytic Quarterly, 26*(3), 303–357.

Renik, O. (2006). *Practical psychoanalysis for therapists and patients.* New York, NY: The Other Press.

Saakvitne, K. (2002). Shared trauma: The therapist's increased vulnerability. *Psychoanalytic Dialogues, 12*(3), 443–449.

Sandler, J. (1976). Countertransference and role responsiveness. *International Review of Psychoanalysis, 3*, 43–47.

Slochower, J. (2003). The analyst's secret delinquencies. *Psychoanalytic Dialogues, 13*(4), 451–469.

Stone, M. (2006). The analyst's body as tuning fork: Embodied resonance in countertransference. *Journal of Analytic Psychology, 51*(1), 109–124.

CHAPTER 7

HEARING THE CRIES OF THE WORLD: THE ROLE OF THERAPISTS' TEARS IN COMPASSION-FOCUSED THERAPY

Dennis Tirch and Laura R. Silberstein

Louis[1]:	When I got back from last weekend at the beach with my friends, I just felt completely shattered. I knew I had to head back into my office and I wanted to die. It was supposed to be a fun weekend, and everyone was so nice to me, but I was terrified of rejection constantly and felt like giving up.
Therapist:	That sounds awful, really. I'm imagining you in the middle of the party, and smiling, but just so scared inside. And, you wanted to die?
Louis:	Well, I didn't really want to die. You don't have to worry about suicide questions and all that stuff. I just felt like giving up. It was awful. I know that the weekend was supposed to be perfect, and we went to a few parties, but all I kept feeling was this intense anxiety and I hated myself for feeling that. What the hell is wrong with me? I am around close friends, and I'm just terrified and I'm sure that they hate me. And when they get closer, I feel it more. How pathetic (Louis is looking downward with tears in his eyes).

(continued)

(continued)

Therapist: *My God, that sounds like a nightmare of a weekend. I'm impressed that you are still engaging in things that matter to you, even though your mind keeps shaming you and telling you that you aren't lovable. It is so hard to carry that around, isn't it?*

Louis: *I know! And it makes me feel crazy and angry. Am I crazy?*

Therapist: *Crazy? This sounds distressing, but it doesn't sound crazy to me at all. It makes so much sense that you would still have these old emotional memories of fear triggered when you are in close relationships, doesn't it? You've told me about so much terrible treatment throughout your childhood, and from people who were very close to you.*

Louis: *Yeah . . . it was . . . it was pretty bad . . . actually, it was very bad (crying quietly).*

Therapist: *It is so very sad, really, to think of you going through that kind of treatment (the therapist is visibly sad around this, but the sadness is contained and tears are not evident). It isn't your fault that you were harmed and treated badly, even abused. If you had let your guard down then, it would have been such a mistake, I think. That's a hard-learned lesson. You didn't choose to learn this kind of fear and to carry this kind of self-criticism. You didn't choose any of it, and it is not your fault.*

Louis: *(pauses as if considering this idea) I know. And it still makes me so angry that nobody protected me, you know? I know that my mother and my sister could hear me being thrown around Dad's office, bouncing off his desk. I know they could hear me yelling. The only time Mom came in was when she heard him repeatedly hitting me in the head with a book! That is so sick to me. I was 12. And I hadn't done anything! I'm so full of hate and sadness right now (Louis is crying now, and he looks up at the therapist).*

Therapist: *You know, Louis, I . . . I am just so sad that anyone could treat that little boy like that, could treat you like that. I am so sorry that you have to know what it is like to feel so hurt and to know what it is like to really hate an abuser, to really hate someone whom you also love. I want you to know that I think it just sucks that you*

> *have been put through this. You have every right to your anger and your sadness (the therapist has visible tears in his eyes at this point and the eye contact and understanding between the therapist and client make the tears of each party known to the other—both are clearly sad, though neither appears out of control).*
>
> **Louis:** *(pausing for a long time and slowing his breathing through the tears) Thank you for actually noticing and actually caring. I didn't know someone would do that. Do you know what it feels like?*
>
> **Therapist:** *I really respect how close you have let me be to your pain and how much you have let yourself share your story here with me. That is brave, Louis. I know these feelings have been here for a long time, and that they will return, like old traveling companions. And, most importantly, they are here, now, with us in the room. It would really matter to me, if we could work together to help you look after yourself, and learn how to feel cared for by others in your life. I know how frightening that can be for you. Do you think you would be willing to work on that here?*
>
> **Louis:** *(crying, but able to speak with a tone of greater warmth and confidence than before) I want to work on that. I feel a lot safer now. I'm sorry.*
>
> **Therapist:** *No need to apologize for feeling here, Louis. We are human. We have emotions, and that is perfectly all right, here and now. I appreciate that you could trust me with these feelings. I know it is a big thing.*
>
> **Louis:** *Yes, it is. I think we can work on this, you know? I really do.*

In this chapter, we will describe the theoretical framework from which I (DT), as Louis' therapist, was practicing. We will also discuss Louis' case, and specifically, the role of the therapist's tears, in more depth. First, we feel it important to mention that whenever we read a case example, it is easy to forget that every example reflects a real person in suffering, just like the many clients we have committed to help, and just like us. In fact, Louis is not an example of a "case" at all, but is an example of an *actual human being*, who carries the same hopes, fears, and sorrows that we all carry. Importantly, this atmosphere of dignity and mutual respect was the perspective from which

I viewed him and related to him. I was practicing a form of evidence-based therapy known as compassion-focused therapy (CFT; Gilbert, 2010).

COMPASSION-FOCUSED THERAPY

Basic Tenets of CFT

Developed by Paul Gilbert in the United Kingdom, CFT is a multimodal psychotherapy approach grounded in affective neuroscience, behavioral research, evolutionary psychology, and the developmental psychology of attachment (Gilbert, 2010). Additionally, many CFT methods are drawn from Buddhist meditation and imagery practices that are thousands of years old, many of which focus on the cultivation of compassion. Indeed, a primary aim of CFT is to intentionally bring the training of compassion into the forefront of therapeutic processes (Gilbert, 2005, 2010). Gilbert (2009) describes compassion as a complex process that emerged from "the caregiver mentality" found in human parental care and child rearing. In CFT, compassion is defined as, "a basic kindness, with deep awareness of the suffering of oneself and of other living things, coupled with the wish and effort to relieve it" (Gilbert, 2009, p. 13).

As part of "compassionate mind training" in the therapeutic setting, CFT emphasizes the activation of affiliative emotions (e.g., emotions of social safeness that emerge in warm, stable, and enduring attachment relationships), promoting focused-flexible awareness and attention (i.e., mindfulness), and broadening the client's range of possible behaviors in response to historically challenging contexts. Such new responses are often learned in the therapeutic relationship, with the therapist's real-time emotional responding serving as a reinforcer. Indeed, the therapist's own presence is an important aspect of "compassionate mind training," as the therapist models a compassionate perspective, and aims to embody the qualities of compassion that the therapy seeks to bring forth, through interactions in the therapeutic alliance. In this way, the therapist acts as a "compassionate other" whose compassionate responses will over time be internalized by the client.

Another aspect of cultivating compassion in CFT is the realization, made explicit by the CFT therapist, that we emerge from the flow of life as an evolved being on this planet, as only one version of ourselves, facing life's challenges and tragedies, and that it is *not our fault* (Gilbert, 2009). So many of the challenges we face are not of our choosing and are not our fault. We do not choose our ancestors or parents, nor do we choose the place and circumstances of our birth. We do not choose our economic or cultural circumstances. CFT emphasizes that, by way of these circumstances that are not of our choosing, we often arrive for therapy with well-learned but ineffective ways of responding to suffering and perceived threats. While the challenges we face are not our fault, CFT emphasizes that we can choose to be responsible for finding new ways to answer our life's challenges and deal with our suffering. In this way, CFT seeks to de-shame and de-pathologize human suffering, letting go of self-blame while seeking to take responsibility for directing the course of our lives. To do so, the therapist and the client co-create an emotional atmosphere of social safeness and connectedness that serves an emotion regulation function. Specifically, affiliative emotions down-regulate the excessive activation of threat-focused processing that typically leads to narrowing of attention and behavioral repertoires. In the transcript from Louis' case that opened this chapter, my overtly caring and de-pathologizing stance, as evidenced by my crying, created an environment of safeness and connectedness that allowed Louis to stay with his own difficult experience, something that his old ways of dealing with such difficult feelings had not allowed him to do.

In this way, CFT asks therapists to do more than to work on the level of changing propositional knowledge structures through rational disputation and altering cognitions. By deliberately drawing upon the functioning of our compassionate mind, we are activating our capacity for genuine empathy and deeply felt sympathy, training in ourselves an innate capacity for effective emotion regulation. In technical terms, CFT therapists engage in empathic bridging and affect matching, wherein they deliberately extend flexible perspective-taking to actively imagine what it would be like to experience the client's experience. Furthermore, when verbally validating or reflecting upon the client's experience, a CFT therapist is encouraged to match some of the affect that the client feels and express the emotions that he or she is feeling in response. Of course, such a therapist is going to be deeply moved by the client's emotions, and when appropriate, the therapist may even be brought to tears by the client's suffering. Attempts to short-circuit the slightest release of tears could effectively hinder this empathic process.

Evolutionary Psychology, CFT, and Crying

As we mentioned above, one important aspect of CFT is its focus on evolutionary psychology. When we recognize the impact of evolution—a process over which we as individuals have no control—on the current state of our minds and bodies, we can become more compassionate toward the ways that our minds and bodies behave (i.e., the emotions and responses they produce that sometimes cause us great distress). Our bodies and brains are the current outcome of evolutionary processes involving natural selection, as described by multilevel selection theory (Buss, 2009; Cortina & Liotti, 2014; Panksepp, 2010). Thus, we each have a human brain and body shaped by millions of years of slow adaptation to changing contexts with a focus on enhancing the chance of survival of ourselves, our species, and our genetic inheritance. Having to continually build upon the previous design, evolution leaves us today with brains and bodies that contain systems and functions that are found across a variety of species. This evolutionary perspective provides us with a basis for understanding how our brains were formed and how they influence our minds and experience (Buss, 2009; Gilbert, 2001, 2007, 2009; Panksepp, 1998). In this section, we will discuss the evolution of compassion and crying in humans.

Human infants are born defenseless, and at a low birth rate. Infant survival in this situation is supremely important and our offspring require a great deal of care and protection in order to survive. About 150 million years ago we see the emergence of certain mammalian brain structures and elements of the nervous and hormonal systems that support nurturing, caregiving, and protective behaviors (Gilbert, 2010). This is evolution's response to the vulnerable nature of our offspring. In fact, a large array of caregiving and nurturing behaviors can be observed throughout mammalian species, including the human species. Humans' capacity for compassion evolved as an extension of the mammalian attachment system and its related motives and abilities for caring for others (Bowlby, 1969; Wang, 2005). Humans have evolutionary advantages compared to all other species that also contribute to our capacity for compassion. These unique capacities include cognition, cooperation, self-awareness, and the ability to base complex behaviors on abstract processes such as thought, imagery, and feeling (Tirch, Schoendorff & Silberstein, 2014). Thus, human compassion is theorized to have emerged from an evolutionarily determined "species-preservative" neurophysiological system (Wang, 2005). This "species-preservative" system is younger in evolutionary terms than the "self-preservative" systems that exists in many other species. Wang (2005) asserts that this newer system is based on an "inclusive sense of self and promotes awareness of our interconnectedness to others" (p. 75). The human prefrontal cortex, cingulate cortex, and the ventral vagal complex are suggested to be factors in the activation of the "species-preservative" system. Importantly, for our purposes, these brain and nervous system structures are all involved in developing healthy attachment bonds and self-compassion (Gilbert, 2009). We have evolved with a capacity to down-regulate excessive threat detection through the activation of affiliative emotions and compassion, and this has important implications for the relevance of therapists' crying in therapy.

Let us now examine crying from the perspective of an evolutionary functional analysis of behavior to highlight potential functions of our tears. Hasson and Unit (2009) suggest that crying serves a number of important functions in the context of human interpersonal relationships. The blurring of vision, loss of muscle tone, and overall vulnerability that we arrive in when we cry may serve as a behavioral signal that we are non-threatening to other members of our family or group. This may function as a submissive display, signaling that others are safe to approach. Importantly, this also may function as a signal of distress and that help is needed. Tears may have served the function of generating sympathy and/or eliciting actual help from a group member in a time of emotional pain or crisis. The vulnerability signaled by crying may also serve the function of provoking some form of mercy or at least a cessation of hostility in an aggressor. The sum of the global research has suggested that crying conveys a message that there is a need for attachment and bonding, that it is safe to approach, and that crying can enhance a shared attachment bond (Hasson & Unit, 2009). The intimacy of shared vulnerability that occurs during crying contributes to a context of social safeness that is essential in human emotion regulation and subsequent effective action. Accordingly, crying is intimately connected to the activation of compassion as conceptualized within the CFT model.

Crying is a highly evolved human behavior and, as far as we know, humans are the only animals that cry for purely emotional reasons. Importantly, our tears are only likely to be seen by people who are nearby, revealing the extent of our distress and the degree to which we are moved by our emotions only to our most intimate companions (Vingerhoets & Cornelius, 2001). Tears might let others close to us know that we need help, without revealing the extent of our vulnerability to potential predators or adversaries. So, when Louis and I both could see one another's tears, and Louis was aware that he was being looked after and protected in the context of the psychotherapeutic relationship, we can imagine that the minds of both parties were activating an intersubjective matrix of compassion that could facilitate growth and change.

Importantly, our tears are triggered not only by sadness, but by a range of human emotions. Physical pain, grief, rage, frustration, and even joy can all lead us to tears. When we see a person in tears, we are immediately aware of that individual's emotional state, or at least we are aware that the person's emotions have significantly affected his or her state of being. As a result, our capacity for flexible perspective-taking and empathic responding is triggered and potentiated by our experience of another person crying. This capacity for empathy likely played an important role in the human evolutionary advantage of being an "ultra-cooperative" species (Cortina & Liotti, 2014). Noting that crying appears to elicit compassion, Povinelli, Bering, and Giambrone (2000) suggest that human relationships have been facilitated and preserved by our capacity for tears. When infants cry, their needs and distress become evident to all people within range of hearing. Accordingly, our evolutionary infant ancestors who were able to cry and thus elicit assistance and command attention were more likely to have their needs met by their parents and other members of their group, and were less likely to find themselves abandoned to the mercy of strangers.

Compassion and Crying

Let us return for a moment to CFT's roots in the long-standing tradition of Buddhist meditation. For centuries, global wisdom traditions have taught that consciously training the mind in compassion, through mindfulness and imagery practices which CFT actively incorporates, could have abundant benefits for personal well-being and growth. Our English term "compassion" comes from a Latin root (*com-patio*) that means "suffering with." Furthermore, the historical name of the archetypal Buddhist personification of compassion (the Bodhisattva of Compassion Avilokiteshvara (Pali) or Kannon-Bosatsu (Japanese)) can be translated as "The One Who Hears the Cries of the World." It seems that our intellectual ancestors in pre-scientific traditions were aware of the healing power of an empathic resonance that allows us to experience the crying and suffering of our fellow humans as if it were our own, leading us to share in their suffering, motivating us to take action. From such a perspective, therapists' tears in psychotherapy sessions can be an aspect of a significant compassionate motivation that can directly lead to committed action to alleviate and prevent suffering, on the part of both the therapist and the client.

THERAPISTS' TEARS IN CFT

If you were to meet Louis, you would likely be impressed. Impeccably dressed, and hailing from a trendy neighborhood in New York, he has a seemingly effortless ability to project a sense of style, and exhibits a wry sense of humor that suggests a deep cultural fluency, keen intelligence, and a joy in living. Louis works for an internet-marketing start-up, always remaining current with developments in technology and up to date on just about every aspect of life that a millennial entrepreneur might be expected to embrace. Despite the social currency of all of these signifiers, Louis has been secretly living in shame and pain. His inner dialogue has been relentlessly harsh and cruelly self-evaluative for many years. Since his adolescence, he has endured persistent flashbacks to repeated childhood trauma and abuse.

As he began his therapy, Louis' desire for relief from this suffering was intense, and he was motivated to take the steps necessary for change. During the course of his therapy with one of the authors (DT), Louis repeatedly aimed to implement a range of cognitive and behavioral strategies that he had learned for dealing with anxiety, self-criticism, and traumatic re-experiencing. He was a quick study. Though he did make some progress in symptom reduction using methods gleaned from the "gold standard" of evidence-based psychotherapies, he continued to struggle with deeply painful and shame-based personal perceptions for a good portion of his therapy.

Over time in working with me (DT), Louis was gradually able to find a way of accepting, containing, and working with his difficult emotions and memories. Rather than simply "getting rid" of his unwanted thoughts and feelings, he described eventually developing a "new capacity" for accepting them in the course of his therapy. This new "psychic muscle" (as he described it) grew with his ability to meet his experience with present-moment-focused awareness, hold himself in kindness, and consciously direct compassion towards himself. He gained these abilities through training in mindfulness, compassion-focused imagery practice, responding with compassion and warmth to his negative thoughts and destructive emotions, and, importantly, through his actual experience of compassion and empathy from me which, in turn, shaped his behavior naturalistically in the therapeutic relationship. This process of developing Louis' "psychic muscle" seemed to begin in earnest during a session when both he and I were brought to tears by the weight of the suffering and rage Louis had been carrying, the transcript of which began this chapter. Far from being an obstacle to therapy, Louis described his experience of my tears in therapy as reflective of our significant connection, an honest validation, and a real emotional resonance that served as a platform for personal growth. For Louis, my tears and emotional self-disclosure served as a powerful social reinforcer that shaped his capacity for self-compassion.

As we described in discussing the basic tenets of CFT above, an important role of the CFT therapist is to engage in empathic bridging and affect matching. In the case of Louis, the intensity of rage and sadness that Louis expressed when he described his experience at the beach with his friends triggered in me a sympathetic sadness and a compassionate urge to help Louis better bear the suffering he was carrying. Rather than turning away from my powerful emotional response, I examined and verbalized what was moving us both to tears. There was a great deal of information in this response. More than simply "feeling bad" for Louis, I felt a personal sadness. This sadness emerged naturally from the realization that the young man sitting across from me had so much of his life experience colored by a deep hatred and expectation of rejection. I actually felt grief for the years that Louis had lost to fear of rejection, anticipation of abuse, and persistent self-criticism. It is sad to imagine someone you care about going through that kind of pain, and Louis was someone whom I cared about. Rather than hiding this response, or diverting my focus to attempts at experiential avoidance, I spoke empathically from this grief, and Louis was receptive to what was being said. He was given clear proof of my genuine compassion and empathic awareness through both my tears and my words, but more importantly, he became engaged by the clarity and wisdom that accompany authentic and unfiltered empathic perspective-taking.

In addition to expressing the grief I felt for Louis, my tears expressed another sadness—sadness for others like Louis. When I said to Louis, "I am just so sad that anyone could treat that little boy like that, could treat you like that," I was talking about "that little boy" that was Louis, but was also any child who has endured terrible pain in circumstances that are not of his or her choosing or fault. In this sense, while our shared tears connected Louis and me in his suffering, they also connected us to a larger suffering, a common humanity: they helped us to "hear the cries of the world." This connection and enhanced perspective-taking regarding our own suffering in relation to the suffering of others can be profoundly healing and hopeful.

As a result, my tears carried a great deal of reinforcing value. Crying, in this case, did not signify emotional dysregulation, but communicated some of the most important evolutionary messages that adult tears convey. The tears told Louis that I understood him, that I was moved by his suffering, that this was a context of social safeness, and that the interaction between us contained honesty, and a motivation to share and work with difficult emotions and challenges. The tears also helped us both feel a sense of connection to a greater human suffering that is not our fault, but is part of a life that we all, in some way, endure. This did not in any way minimize the suffering Louis experienced but, quite the opposite, allowed us to understand and appreciate his suffering as something that connected him to—as opposed to isolated him from—others. Indeed, part of cultivating self-compassion is cultivating a sense of common humanity: instead of seeing one's own suffering as a problem with oneself or as isolating—as Louis felt about his anxiety—one begins to see suffering as part of the human condition, something that connects us all. The tears a therapist cries are, in and of themselves, a sign of this shared humanity: I cry for Louis, I share his suffering. My tears are proof of our human condition.

Louis' case is a useful example to discuss therapist tears because Louis actively commented on our shared crying. In the beginning of the session following my crying, Louis thanked me for an important session the prior week. He said that when he noticed his mind engaging in cruel or self-critical dialogue during the week since our session, he remembered me speaking to him with tears in my eyes, and would imagine what I would say in response to the self-criticism. He used this imagery to generate compassionate self-statements that he then wrote into his iPhone's "notes" app, so that he could be reminded of them later. Louis and I continued to use these experiences to help him build a range of responses from an imaginary "compassionate other" that he actively related to during advanced mindful compassion imagery exercises and active inner dialogue. When this case was discussed with experienced CFT therapists in peer supervision, including both of the authors of this chapter and the CFT founder, Paul Gilbert, the consensus of the discussion was that my tears created the context for the client's learning and internalizing empathy, sensitivity, and a motivation to care. Importantly, the shared crying while persisting in valued directions allowed Louis to experience and rehearse distress tolerance and resilience that he could draw upon later in real time.

CONCLUSION AND RECOMMENDATIONS

During the therapy session with Louis that opened this chapter, Louis explicitly told me that it mattered to him that I cared enough to be moved to tears about his abuse, and also felt gratified that I trusted him enough to show tears without hiding. If a therapist is able to maintain sufficient composure and affect regulation to continue the dialogue with his or her client, and also is directing his or her focus towards the client's emotions rather than being diverted to the therapist's own needs or losing him- or herself in an immersive experience of his or her own distress and crying, then there is no need for the therapist to actively suppress tears. Indeed, research shows that withholding one's emotions can seriously hinder interactions with others (Van Kleef, 2009). Furthermore, there is no specific diagnosis or problem set to which this openness and compassion should be limited. Of course, it is important that the therapist's response remains matched to the affective intensity and valence of the client's experience, or there could be a bizarre disconnection.

Just as CFT teaches clients to respond to their emotional experiences in the present moment with mindfulness and self-compassion, the CFT therapist does not deploy any specific skills to manage or "cope" with the feelings that might result in therapist crying in session. Rather, the CFT therapist meets this experience with mindful compassion, affording the training that allows us to maintain psychological flexibility and engage in compassionate action as a therapist even during emotional experiences that prompt tears.

Indeed, while there are a few existing therapy models that base their rationale on the importance of empathy and the literature on the affect-regulating function of secure attachment bonds, CFT alone places the cultivation of compassion at the center of the psychotherapy agenda. This training of the compassionate mind (for both client and therapist) takes place in a variety of ways, including: practice of techniques that facilitate mindfulness and relaxation; systematic training of compassion-focused imagery exercises; self-help cognitive reappraisal methods drawing upon a compassionate perspective; modeling of the compassionate mind in the psychotherapy relationship; shaping compassionate responding through social reinforcement in the therapeutic alliance; and compassion-focused behavioral change methods, including exposure and response prevention and behavioral activation. In this modality, the therapist's genuine emotional responding and affect matching of the client's emotional state are both central therapist microskills and explicit techniques. Accordingly, the therapist's tears in therapy are a useful, naturalistically arising tool for the internalization and cultivation of compassionate responding, resilience, and psychological flexibility. The qualities that emerge with our evolved compassionate mentality include a sense of courage, wisdom, and authority. If a therapist is simultaneously tearful and embodying the emotional intelligence of the compassionate mind, the benefits of such authenticity and embodied compassion can assuage any potential fears of tears.

NOTE

1. All potentially identifying details of the client's life, as well as aspects of the transcript, have been modified to preserve anonymity and privacy.

REFERENCES

Bowlby, J. (1969). *Attachment.* New York, NY: Basic Books.
Buss, D. M. (2009). The great struggles of life: Darwin and the emergence of evolutionary psychology. *American Psychologist, 64,* 140–148.

Cortina, M., & Liotti, G. (2014). An evolutionary outlook on motivation: Implications for the clinical dialogue. *Psychoanalytic Inquiry*, *34*(8), 864–899.

Gilbert, P. (2001). Evolutionary approaches to psychopathology: The role of natural defences. *Australian and New Zealand Journal of Psychiatry*, *35*, 17–27.

Gilbert, P. (Ed.). (2005). *Compassion: Conceptualizations, research and use in psychotherapy*. New York, NY: Routledge.

Gilbert, P. (2007). Evolved minds and compassion in the therapeutic relationship. In P. Gilbert & R. Leahy (Eds.), *The therapeutic relationship in the cognitive behavioral psychotherapies*. New York, NY: Routledge.

Gilbert, P. (2009). *The compassionate mind: A new approach to life's challenges*. London: Constable Robinson.

Gilbert, P. (2010). *Compassion focused therapy: The CBT distinctive features series*. London: Routledge.

Hasson, O., & Unit, B. (2009). Emotional tears as biological signals. *Evolutionary Psychology*, *7*(3), 363–370.

Panksepp, J. (1998). The periconscious substrates of consciousness: Affective states and the evolutionary origins of the self. *Journal of Consciousness Studies*, *5*, 5–6.

Panksepp, J. (2010). Affective neuroscience of the emotional BrainMind: Evolutionary perspectives and implications for understanding depression. *Dialogues in Clinical Neuroscience*, *12*(4), 533.

Povinelli, D. J., Bering, J. M., & Giambrone, S. (2000). Toward a science of other minds: Escaping the argument by analogy. *Cognitive Science*, *24*(3), 509–541.

Tirch, D., Schoendorff, B., & Silberstein, L. R. (2014). *The ACT practitioner's guide to the science of compassion: Tools for fostering psychological flexibility*. Berkeley, CA: New Harbinger.

Van Kleef, G. (2009). How emotions regulate social life: The emotions as social information (EASI) model. *Current Directions in Psychological Science*, *18*(3), 184–188.

Vingerhoets, A. J. J. M., & Cornelius, R. R. (2001). *Adult crying: A biopsychosocial approach*. New York, NY: Brunner-Routledge.

Wang, S. (2005). A conceptual framework for integrating research related to the physiology of compassion and the wisdom of Buddhist teachings. In P. Gilbert (Ed.), *Compassion: Conceptualizations, research and use in psychotherapy*. New York, NY: Routledge.

CHAPTER 8

EXISTENTIAL THERAPY AND THE TRANSFORMATIVE POSSIBILITIES OF THERAPISTS' TEARS

Paul McGinley

I cannot say that I liked Jim.[1] Although he had been regularly attending therapy with me for several months, I was having a hard time connecting with him. He seemed uninterested in self-exploration or revelation—and therefore uninterested in therapy itself—and often had a guarded, condescending, even hostile manner. I suspected that his attendance had more to do with his need to adhere to the court order that brought him to my practice, so as to remain within the benefit system of United Kingdom social services, than any particular commitment to understanding himself.

Jim had been involved in drug use over many years, had never worked and, based on what he related, had been little more than physically present to his family. As far as I could make out from his avoidant account, his daughter, from the age of ten—when she was not rescuing him from the local bar where he was regularly so drunk that he could not find his way home—cooked, cleaned, and kept house, having taken on the role of the mother who herself was addicted to drugs. In spite of taking on these adult responsibilities, she found her way to school—which I imagined was a sort of refuge for her; a place with a sense of order and routine that it seemed unlikely she experienced with her father.

(continued)

> *(continued)*
>
> *Then one morning Jim turned up and seemed unusually engaged. He reported that he had received good news and was celebrating the fact that his daughter, who was now 18, had been accepted at a reputable university where she was going to study.*
>
> *"I am so proud of her. She has really achieved something in her life," Jim said, and he became suddenly tearful. This was the first time I had experienced what I understood as a sense of humanity in Jim or an acknowledgment of anyone other than himself. I felt a resonance in myself; I connected with what I thought was a shared sense of awe at his daughter, an acknowledgment of her strength, resilience, and endurance. Indeed, I felt connected to Jim for the first time, and tears came to my eyes as I joined him in his validation. Then, as if out of the blue, he said, "It makes me realize that I've done a pretty good job."*
>
> *I felt caught in a lie. The shared understanding that I had assumed in Jim's tears, and which had resonated in me, turned out to be Jim taking credit for his daughter's achievement, despite the fact that, for all I could apprehend, she had achieved this in spite of what he had put her through. I felt my tears had somehow validated Jim's own interpretation and that I had been caught up in a dynamic where my own feelings had been confiscated and now seemed fraudulent to myself.*

In this chapter, I will discuss the issues raised in this example from an existential perspective, with particular reference to self-disclosure, transparency, responsibility, self-identity, and transformation. Before doing so, I will briefly describe the understanding of existential psychotherapy that informs my work and my understanding of the nature and meaning of tears.

EXISTENTIAL PSYCHOTHERAPY AND TEARS

Basic Tenets of Existential Psychotherapy

Existential psychotherapy is a broad church encompassing a number of different strands, both in terms of ontological commitments and methodological approaches. Although there have been, and continue to be, enthusiastic attempts to delineate and define existential therapy as a unique modality in its own right, I would suggest that it is, at heart, a manner of approach informed by philosophy and characterized by an overall concern for who we are and how we are to live, rather than an adherence to any particular theory. Indeed, many existential psychotherapists are averse to both theories and any "tools" that may arise from them.

Some writers trace the roots of existential psychotherapy to Søren Kierkegaard (van Deurzen, 1997, 2002) whilst others would suggest that they go as far back as the Ancient Greeks in the thought of Anaximander, Parmenides, and Heraclitus (Heaton, 2003). The latter is not surprising when we consider that existential psychotherapy is focused on the human condition and, therefore, its concerns have been with us as long as human beings have existed. Given this enormously broad terrain, it should come as no surprise that there is a great deal of diversity and complexity within the existential therapeutic community. In this chapter, I will focus on the major characteristics of existential thought and practice that are most relevant to the subject of crying.

Two distinct strands underlie existential psychotherapy. One—made popular by Sartre (1989) in the public psyche following the upheavals of World War II—holds that the world is fundamentally meaningless, and that it is our task therefore to *create* meaning for ourselves, and furthermore that we are all isolated individuals attempting, with greater or lesser success, to find ways to relate to others. There is, however, another strand, which holds that we always already dwell within a world *saturated* with meanings that we are constantly engaged in revealing, and that we are always related to others at a fundamental level—albeit that such relatedness is realized in many different ways, some more appropriate and fulfilling than others. Personally, I come from this latter position and believe, following Heidegger's (1962) concept of "being-in-the-world," that we are always already related and furthermore, that we are most ourselves when we are engaged in the process of revealing the meaning of our relatedness to the world and others.

What remains constant across any variations and conceptual differences between existential psychotherapists, however, is the understanding that human beings differ from other kinds of beings in that we *know* we exist, and furthermore, that we *care* about our existence, i.e., that our existence is an issue for us (Heidegger, 1962). It follows that existential psychotherapists are concerned with the exploration of beliefs, values, and purpose, i.e., the *meaning* of people's lives.

Where such meaning is located is debated within the existential therapeutic community. Whilst some existential psychotherapists hold that meaning exists primarily at a cognitive level (indeed, being "philosophical" has taken on connotations of disembodiment, and cognitive emphasis), where our affective response is informed by our rational, or sometimes irrational, interpretations of events, others take a different view in holding that what we feel is already an intelligible response to a situation that can then be further articulated and understood at a cognitive level. Whatever position existential therapists take with regard to the primacy of cognition or affect, what is common to *all* is that there is no final authority to whom we can turn to tell us how to respond to the meanings we find in the world.[2] Therefore, we are faced with the challenge to accept, reject, incorporate, or re-evaluate the values and meanings already given to us (or to hold by ones that we believe we have created for ourselves). Either way, we are confronted with the ultimate question of *ownership*, commonly thought of in terms of responsibility, i.e., the challenge to *respond* to the situations we find ourselves thrown into but did not explicitly choose. The aim and project of existential psychotherapy therefore, rather than being concerned with agendas of change, help, or improvement, are primarily characterized by the enterprise of revealing, exploring, and understanding the meanings in someone's life, allowing for the possibility of greater self-responsibility.

Whilst understanding the human way of being has been, and continues to be, the concern of philosophy as well as the arts, the element that sets existential psychotherapy aside from these other disciplines is that its endeavor is attempted through the phenomenological method. Phenomenology means, in short, bringing things to light.[3] This method is primarily defined by the attempt to see a phenomenon freshly, unencumbered by assumptions or traditional conceptualizations that overlie and cover up original lived experience. This uncovering of original meaning applies just as much to the everyday language that we use, which is characterized by euphemisms that hide more than they reveal, as it does to more formal academic theories that are often based on assumptions about the human way of being that the person adhering to them is not aware.

The extent to which we are able to bring our own ways of being to light, and thereby own or disown them, is the degree to which we can say that we are authentically being ourselves. Authenticity, then, is not based upon any particular action or belief, but on the extent to which we are able to take responsibility for the actions and behaviors we find ourselves performing.[4] This, of course, is closely related to what it means to be authentically with another, which brings us to the heart of the challenge of therapists' tears in therapy.

Having laid out this brief outline of existential psychotherapy, I will now discuss my understanding of the nature of tears, the challenge that tears bring to our understanding of authenticity, and how that is played out in the therapeutic project.

Tears: An Existential Framework

> Though I know not what is enshrined, my tears flow in the face of its awesomeness.
>
> (*Sankashū*, Saigyō, 1179/1991)

Perspective, ambiguity, surface, and depth; the precarious stability of maintaining a sense of self; these are but some of the issues forefronted and exposed in the phenomenon of crying. Generally, little is said about these matters, and what is spoken of tears is often marred in euphemisms, such as "breaking down," "falling apart," or "getting upset," that overlie the primordial challenge that crying brings as it occurs in the therapeutic encounter.

To achieve an appropriate relationship with any phenomenon, it is helpful to have an understanding of what it is—even more so, if we can understand what it is in its essence. What is most apparent about crying, and what both motivates and underlies many of the everyday euphemisms that refer to it, is the obvious fact that it is not something we intentionally *do*. It is, rather, something that befalls us, or overcomes us—to deliberately cry would suggest manipulative "crocodile tears."

What can be said of it, then, is that the essence of crying lies in the fact that it speaks from an otherness within us that is both us, and not us. But, because this phenomenon occurs before, in spite of, and *in excess* of any intention, it becomes an interlocutor in a conversation between who I think I am and who I may be. Once understood in this way, my tears do not just bring cathartic relief, but rather, seen in light of what they show me, reverberate across the perceived expanse between my sense of self and the world of the other as both a challenge and a call. In a situation of authentic crying, the condition of which can never be of my own making, the phenomenon acts to both disclose my affective life to myself, as well as to fill the perceived gap between me, and the other.

But how is such a gap filled? Tears do not appear to us in the way other objects do; indeed, they do not appear to us as objects at all because, undermining the assumed split between the material body and the psyche, they are always already imbued with existential significance as both a demand and an appeal; the appearance of tears is not the same as water dripping from a tap, they require a response both from ourselves and the other.[5] Therefore, in speaking of "tears" we are already moving within a conceptual framework structured in terms of existential meanings, rather than material objects. As Heidegger states in *Zollikon Seminars* (2001):

> You can never actually measure tears. If you try to measure them, you measure a fluid and its drops at the most, but not tears. Tears can only be seen directly. Where do tears belong? Are they something somatic or psychical? They are neither the one, nor the other.
>
> (Heidegger, 2001, p. 81)

What is in these tears that we cry, and what would their accomplishment be? For some, such as clients I can think of, allowing oneself to cry is itself the task, whilst for others it is experienced as their ruin. But from a phenomenological perspective, this question must be understood as a fundamental challenge of ownership through a process of adoption and appropriation. The phenomenological experience of crying, if allowed to be what it is, has a dialogical nature: it is both speaking and being spoken to, being held and yet opened up, calling and being called, tamed and released to abandon. The understanding of this relational encounter is fundamental to any radical transformation of what it means to be a self, because my interpretation of the meaning of my tears both expresses as well as establishes who I am as an ethical subject. What it demonstrates is that my self is by no means the ego, or self-construct; my self lies in the world within which I dwell and *is* that ethical "being-with-others."

Crying, in line with the ideas put forward in Jack Barbalet's paper, "Weeping and Transformations of Self," can be usefully seen as "an emotional and physical register of changes in self, both positive and negative" (2005, p. 125).[6] However, although crying can be viewed as an *indicator* of a moment of reinterpretation of oneself, within such a conceptualization Barbalet falls back on the idea that crying "is a predominantly *physical* [emphasis added] engagement of a self that is involved in non-symbolic interior communication" (Barbalet, 2005, p. 134). Here, he fails to read the ontological significance of crying, in that we are confronted with a phenomenon that invites a Copernican revolution (Todres, 1997) where the locus of meaning no longer resides in *us* (and certainly not in our cognitive evaluations), but rather in our existence "in-the-world," which is prior to who we think we may be. I will say more about this below to clarify this point.

TEARS IN THERAPY

The emergence of crying by the therapist is often understood to be an empathic reflection of others' suffering through which our humanity emerges above and beyond the therapeutic role. Whilst this seems to be correct enough, from my perspective, being transparent to our clients in who we are, being authentic in our response, not adopting an exaggerated attitude of empathy towards the other, or hiding what we truly feel, is already assumed, and is not something that only becomes expressed in moments such as crying—not least because such occurrences always contain the possibility of solipsistic self-interest. Rather, as I understand it, crying speaks to an experience of *participation* in the human condition that is others', yours, and mine, and that has a communal dimension that blurs and broaches the boundaries between the individuals with and through whom it comes.

Due to its inherently relational nature, understanding my own affective response is a fundamental aspect of existential psychotherapy as I practice it; being sensitive to what I am experiencing in response to this other is important for understanding my client's relational world. Following from this, questions around what to do with such understanding (e.g., questions related to self-disclosure and transparency, both essential concerns in the challenge of therapists' tears) inevitably arise.

In order to get clearer about these matters it may be helpful to define what we *mean* by self-disclosure. I do not readily share my personal circumstances and details with clients, and when I do, in line with other existential psychotherapists (Spinelli, 1989, 1994), I feel it has to fulfill two criteria. Firstly, that the matter has arisen out of what is being discussed and seems relevant to what is happening in the session and therefore has not been randomly introduced by me—in this way, disclosure contextualizes my own particular interpretation and perspective on the matter, as well as hopefully offering some illumination on the subject. Secondly, that sharing a particular piece of information may have therapeutic value that outweighs what could otherwise be an imposition upon the client's space. This second "rule" is, of course, always difficult to judge, and one can never be sure.

Where self-disclosure takes on a different meaning, however, is in the transparency that one allows in terms of affective response. Here, in line with my understanding of existential psychotherapy, I would rarely attempt to hide or cover up what I am feeling in response to the other (i.e., my client). The rationale for this lies primarily in the existential concept of "being-with" (Heidegger, 1962), which holds that we are always already with others, despite sometimes hiding away or avoiding them. Therefore, bringing our way of being with the client to light, i.e., doing phenomenology on the relationship that is always already there, is an important aspect of what is therapeutic in existential psychotherapy. In fact, I would hold that there is an ethical imperative to such disclosure, even when that might demand difficult things being said.[7] The challenge, therefore, with regard to allowing tears to be transparently seen in psychotherapy does not lie in deciding whether to hide, suppress, or contain them in face of the other, but rather in understanding the *meaning* of those tears, and our responsibility with regard to them.

Within an ethical therapeutic encounter, there is no possibility of conceptualizing, and hence constituting, others' tears as objects of perception (Marion, 2002) without diminishing and concretizing their expansive and fluid sense—simply because any meaning expressed in crying is always beyond, and in excess of, the other's intentionality. Therefore, crying can only be responded to as an injunction that, prior to any attempt to explain it, has already taken the initiative; where tears elude the possibility of being perceived as objects to be looked at but, rather, emerge as a process intimately including the other.[8] But this, of course, must be equally correct of the otherness of our own tears, because authentic tears are necessarily in excess of our *own* intention.

As an existential psychotherapist, I understand part of my role as facilitating my clients' understanding and facing of their issues, and thereby hopefully helping clients to resolve them.[9] But to do this I first need to understand the person, and I believe that to *really* understand another is to be prepared to enter into a dynamic relationship with that other—or, more accurately, to do phenomenology on the relationship with the other that we already find ourselves within, thereby allowing it to develop more deeply. By meeting in this way, we gain access to, and potentially understand, those primordial levels—such as moods, affects, and embodied intelligence—that are prior to, but nevertheless inform and influence, the conceptual, cognitive, evaluative rationality required when deciding upon different actions and choosing which paths to take.

From an existential understanding, we are in no way to be thought of as self-encapsulated beings, but rather as a kind of process; a process that is utterly grounded in our relatedness with others and is, in fact, constituted by it. It is for this reason that Merleau-Ponty is able to state that, "[We] cannot be transparent to ourselves, so that our contact with ourselves is necessarily achieved only in the sphere of ambiguity" (1962, p. 381), because we only find out who we are in relation to the otherness of others. What is less frequently noticed, however, is not the otherness of the other, but the *otherness in us* that comes to light through tears.

In light of this, how are we to make sense of the example given at the beginning of this chapter?

Tears With Jim

Returning now to the case that began this chapter, one could easily suggest that there are different phenomena lying within the overall manifestation of

Jim's tears. One could, for instance, theorize that above and beyond Jim's own interpretation of his tears there lay attachment issues that he was either denying or completely unaware of. Such interpretations have value and are certainly meaningful, but my concern here is to point to the way that tears illuminate our ontological status. Because, as an occasion for dialogue between the cognitive province and a realm of understanding that *feels* the world, the emergence of tears is precisely the beginning of a multi-voiced discussion.

My initial response to Jim's tears was a genuine sense of connection to Jim as another human being whose affective world had opened up. The fact that he appeared to initially understand this in terms of his own achievement is secondary to the fact that the tears had occurred. My sense of my own response having been defrauded was by no means in light of the fact that Jim had cried, but that he had interpreted his crying as primarily *for himself*. However, in order to "work through" such tensions, it is necessary to open oneself up to the humanity of the occurrence of these tears in the first place. By being open and transparent, not only in terms of having allowed my tears to be seen, but in exploring their meaning together with Jim, we found that we were able to establish a level of respect for each other over and above any disagreement in terms of the values we hold.

My intervention, which is not an unusual one for me to make, was to ask Jim what sense *he* made of *my* tears: What did he think they were saying? What was it like for him to experience them? How did they make him feel?

By openly allowing my affective world to be expressed, I was confronting Jim's self-encapsulated sense of himself, as well as modeling a way to be-with one's own affective world. This was a challenge to Jim to acknowledge that he was in relation to me, and others, and respond to the fact that, within therapeutic boundaries, I cared about his daughter as well as about him. Such an intervention also invited Jim to be sensitive to, and access, his own felt response to tears from an optimal distance that was safe enough for him to do so. Rather than talking about relationships in a cognitive fashion, such exploration is a challenge to experience relationships in a *felt* and experiential way, and to develop the ability to understand and express one's own affective responses. Whose tears were these after all? Were they just mine, or were they perhaps Jim's as well, or even his daughter's?

The exploration of the meaning of my crying allowed Jim to explore the meaning of tears more deeply, whereby his understanding of his own was inevitably transformed. Although there was still a sense of Jim's own gratification in his tears, there was also, we discovered, a genuine sense of relief from a burden of responsibility as a parent that he had never felt able to rise up to, but had not felt safe enough to acknowledge. Although he initially interpreted his tears in terms of narcissistic satisfaction, in fact, as we analyzed them more closely, it became clear that there was much more in them than that.[10]

As tears are always already both our own and others', by being open and exploring the meaning of both Jim's tears, and mine, we were able to compare the kind of care that he had received in his own upbringing and the kind that he had offered his daughter, in relation to that experienced in this moment with and from me. In this way, our new understanding of tears also bridged and transformed our relationship to one another. While this process was challenging for Jim at an affective level, it was also transformative; it ultimately offered an opportunity for Jim to relate and respond both to himself and to another human being in ways that he had not previously been open to; to both receive genuine care as well as to find the resource to begin to care for himself. I believe that from such a position it might then be possible to care for others.[11]

But no such exploration would have been possible had we begun from the perspective that these tears—Jim's or my own—arose in response to a cognitive understanding, because from such a position they are already relegated to nothing more than a particularly intense expression of something we already know. Whereas, if we recognize that crying is precisely *unintentional*, then we have to face the fact that it is a form of understanding that is *different* than cognition, is no less significant, and in fact knows something at the level of experience where the word "know" means something other than being propositionally correct.

For although we may be receptive to our tears, and while within such hermeneutic reception we necessarily play a part in rendering them meaningful, we are never actually the authors of the meaning of our crying—in the Sartrean (1989) sense mentioned above, of choosing the values to throw over the phenomenon—not least because, more than any other behavior (if we can use such an ambiguous word in reference to crying),[12] the experience always already precedes any such interpretations. We are only the passive receptors of our crying, and therefore, more than being speaking beings, we are beings that are spoken.

A healing of the separation between will and being—between the way we want to act and how we find ourselves behaving—may only be possible through remaining open to the revelation that crying offers, such that the gap between intention and meaning inherent in this split begins to close as we navigate our way through the labyrinth of our affective lives. Although Jim's tears were primarily for himself, the affective response was itself genuine and was eventually understood and owned by both of us as a participation in the suffering of all others, including his daughter (whose suffering Jim had previously been reluctant to acknowledge) and Jim himself (whose suffering I had previously had a difficult time connecting with). It may be that it was only possible through such engagement with tears, both his and mine, that his way of being—revealed through his affective world of tears[13]—could be understood, and transformed.

CONCLUSIONS AND RECOMMENDATIONS

There are perhaps few such significant moments in psychotherapy as when crying emerges between two people. Whatever else may be said, it is a phenomenon demanding to be noticed. I would not normally hide my felt response and I often ask my clients what sense they make of what it is I am feeling. Such phenomenological clarification is a fundamental part of existential psychotherapy.

I believe it is helpful to keep in mind the primary challenge of tears, which is not what they signify, but the way that they do essentially signify something; that there is a level of understanding here that is above and beyond propositional calculation—we are brought face to face with an ontology of meaning in which we are in no way transparent to ourselves.[14] Therefore, the phenomenon comes to us from an otherness that is deeply within us but which is not, and perhaps never can be, part of us. A part of us that we do not own, that therefore is not our own, is not our property. For that reason it is *im*proper; a fault at the core of our being. It is precisely through this faultline that tears challenge and highlight the vanity of attempting to comprehend that upon which we are ourselves dependent and, in this way, tears are symptomatic of the fact that we are, as Augustine says, "mysterious, even to ourselves" (Rist, 1994, p. 88). Having said that, although tears are an expression of our own lack of transparency to ourselves, they also offer the opportunity of a self-understanding that goes far beyond cognitive self-reflection, and thereby they offer the possibility, as in Jim's case, of freeing us from the limitations of our narcissistic and self-encapsulated constructs.

That said, existential psychotherapy is a way of being rather than any sort of technique or skill set. Training in this modality is focused on the responsibility of the trainee to be the kind of person who may be able to genuinely be with another and therefore it would be disingenuous of me to offer specific recommendations for practice with regard to tears. However, if anything that has been written here challenges, or enriches, a reader's own self-understanding, and invites that person to experience the phenomenon of crying anew, then that would be sufficient and in keeping with an existential approach.

NOTES

1. This particular example is a composite of several cases of my own as well as an anecdote kindly shared with me by a participant during my research into crying. The case has been disguised and altered to maintain confidentiality and for the sake of presenting the argument.
2. The ontology underpinning this chapter holds that meaning is not located in either our cognitive or affective response, but is to be found "in-the-world." Here it is important to differentiate between the "world" and the universe; "world" refers to the shared background of intelligible practices within which we dwell, i.e., if a hammer is too heavy for a particular task, the "too heaviness" is not in the hammer, nor is it in my subjective interpretation, it is "in-the-world" (Heidegger, 1962).
3. Phenomenology itself falls into two schools, one being descriptive and the other interpretational (see Gadamer, 2001; Husserl, 1982, 1989).
4. I would argue that this is commensurate with Freud's project of bringing the unconscious to the conscious, which, after all, can mean little other than taking responsibility for who we are.
5. Whether or not we choose to hide ourselves away when we cry, ontologically, we are still with others.
6. Importantly, Barbalet speaks of the significance of crying as the "expression of self-located and self-significant emotional meanings in place of the cognitive and symbolic staples of speech" (2005, p. 134) but, in doing so, does not seem to fully appreciate the ontological significance in understanding our affective world as an intelligible realm of meanings largely independent of our self-interpretations. Nevertheless, Barbalet's paper adds significantly to current theories of crying.
7. Of course, to attempt to *not* disclose at this level is still a disclosure of how one understands and attempts to do psychotherapy.
8. Although not impossible under clinical conditions, it would require a certain artificial distancing to simply "observe" another crying.
9. Existential psychotherapy is, for me, a fundamentally ethical enterprise and ethical dilemmas, by definition, do not have resolutions; at best, they can be endured and confronted, rather than avoided or denied.
10. It should be noted that existential analysis does not have the same meaning as psychodynamic analysis, and is the process of untangling, rather than interpreting from a pre-existing framework.
11. The fact that he had not previously done this was a guilt that Jim might have to carry, but from an existential perspective, in contrast to

a humanistic one, freedom lies in the ability to tolerate being guilty, and existential guilt is the nerve through which we can truly find ourselves.
12. See Merleau-Ponty's *The Structure of Behavior* (1967).
13. Since the introduction of the emotions in the early 1800s, the grammar of tears has become poor in psychological theories (Dixon, 2006), which is why I have referred to our affective life throughout this chapter, rather than to the very questionable category of the emotions.
14. As stated previously, when they are genuine, tears always signify in a way that has nothing to do with intention, for were they to communicate an intentional message, to self or other, they would be manipulative "crocodile tears."

REFERENCES

Barbalet, J. (2005). Weeping and transformations of self. *Journal for the Theory of Social Behaviour, 35*(2), 125–141.

Dixon, T. (2006). *From passions to emotions: The creation of a secular psychological category.* Cambridge: Cambridge University Press.

Gadamer, H. G. (2001). *Truth and method* (2nd ed.) (J. Weinsheimer & D. G. Marshall, Trans.). London: Sheed & Ward. (Original work published 1975.)

Heaton, J. M. (2003). Pyrrhonian scepticism and psychotherapy. *Journal for the Society for Existential Analysis, 14*(1), 32–47.

Heidegger, M. (1962). *Being and time* (J. Maquarrie & E. Robinson, Trans.). Oxford: Blackwell Publishers. (Original work published 1927.)

Heidegger, M. (2001). *Zollikon seminars: Protocols – conversations – letters* (F. Mayr, Trans.). Evanston, IL: Northwestern University Press. (Original work published 1987.)

Husserl, E. (1982). *Ideas pertaining to a pure phenomenology and to a phenomenological philosophy: First book* (F. Kersten, Trans.). Dordrecht: Kluwer. (Original work published (1913).)

Husserl, E. (1989). *Ideas pertaining to a pure phenomenology: Second book studies in the phenomenology of constitution* (R. Rojcewicz & A. Schuwer, Trans.). Dordrecht: Kluwer. (Original work published 1931.)

Marion, J. L. (2002). *In excess: Studies of saturated phenomena* (R. Horner & V. Berraud, Trans.). New York, NY: Fordham University Press. (Original work published 2001.)

Merleau-Ponty, M. (1962). *Phenomenology of perception* (C. Smith, Trans.). New York, NY: Routledge. (Original work published 1945.)

Merleau-Ponty, M. (1967). *The structure of behavior* (A. L. Fisher, Trans.). Boston, MA: Beacon Press. (Original work published 1942.)

Rist, J. (1994). *Augustine: Ancient thought baptized*. Cambridge: Cambridge University Press.

Saigyõ, S. (1991). *Poems of a mountain home* (B. Watson, Trans.). New York, NY: Columbia University Press.

Sartre, J.- P. (1989). *Being and nothingness: An essay on phenomenological ontology* (H. Barnes, Trans.). London: Routledge. (Original work published 1943.)

Spinelli, E. (1989). *The interpreted world: An introduction to phenomenological psychology*. London: Sage.

Spinelli, E. (1994). *Demystifying therapy*. London: Constable.

Todres, L. (1997). *Embodied enquiry: Phenomenological touchstones for research, psychotherapy and spirituality*. Basingstoke, UK: Palgrave Macmillan.

van Deurzen, E. (1997). *Everyday mysteries: Existential dimensions of psychotherapy*. New York, NY: Routledge.

van Deurzen, E. (2002). *Existential counseling and psychotherapy in practice*. London: Sage.

3

THE CLIENTS WITH WHOM WE CRY

CHAPTER 9

THE TEARS OF ABUSE

Maxine Harris

A group of young boys watched as an older woman sat by the water's edge and looked longingly over the outstretched span of water. The waves went on lapping and rising as if they could reach far, far beyond the horizon. As they continued looking, the boys could see a stream of tears flowing down the woman's pale cheeks.

"Whyever is she crying?" asked one of the boys. "It is such a lovely day. There is no reason for tears."

"Perhaps she has lost something very dear," said an especially small boy. "I think her tears are tears of sadness."

"Nonsense!" said a boy who was somewhat older. "Those are tears of frustration and anger. I think she is waiting for her son to come home from a day of fishing and he promised he would not sail too long on the unpredictable sea. She will certainly scold him when he returns because he has made her wait so long."

Then the oldest boy stood up tall and spoke with authority. "Look how she gazes out over the sea. Those are tears of longing. I am sure that she, too, wishes she could sail far from the borders of her tiny village and see the wonders of the world."

(continued)

> *(continued)*
>
> *"All of you are mistaken," said a boy who had been sitting quietly while the others talked. "Those are tears of joy. She feels happy and privileged to live so close to the water and to be able to feel the ocean breezes on her face."*
>
> *As they continued their bickering about the meaning of the woman's tears, the boys watched her rise and walk over the dunes, back into the village.*
>
> *"I suppose we'll never know," said the boy who had been the first to speak. "After all, they are her tears and only she will ever know their true meaning."*

DOING TRAUMA RECOVERY WORK WITH WOMEN[1]

When therapists work with survivors of emotional, sexual, and physical abuse, whether in groups or individually, they frequently find themselves overwhelmed by the raw and powerful stories they hear. Gentle crying is not an unusual event. But, like the boys in the story above, we often witness or experience tears without knowing just what they mean.

Perhaps the best way to understand the many forms of crying experienced by women and their therapists is to listen to the stories of women who have experienced trauma. I have included such stories[2] in this chapter. The stories here are based on personal work, supervision, and training by a group of therapists at Community Connections, a large not-for-profit behavioral/mental health agency in Washington, D.C., that serves over 3,500 women, men, and children who live with mental illness, addiction, abuse, and homelessness. The therapists whose work is represented have taught in over 40 states and have collectively worked with or heard the stories of several thousand women.

The groups and individual work conducted at Community Connections are drawn from an evidence-based model of treatment, Trauma Recovery and Empowerment (Harris, 1998), that leads women through a recovery process involving education about trauma, remembering, and learning skills and strategies for coping—a model that parallels that described by Judith Herman (1992) and others. A word to set the context might be useful.

The development of the Trauma Recovery and Empowerment (Harris, 1998) group model of treatment is based on four core assumptions:

1. Some current dysfunctional behaviors and/or symptoms may have originated as legitimate coping responses to trauma.

2. Women who experienced repeated trauma in childhood were deprived of the opportunity to develop certain skills necessary for adult coping.
3. Trauma severs core connections to one's family, one's community, and ultimately to oneself.
4. Women who have been abused repeatedly feel powerless and unable to advocate for themselves.

(Harris, 1998, p. xiii)

It should also be noted that women who seek services at clinics like Community Connections rarely come in identifying their primary problem as "trauma." Instead they seek help for depression, anxiety, addiction, or for managing a life that seems unbearably out of control and overwhelming. As a result, their stories tell of lives that feel shattered and broken by more than abuse.

And now for the stories.

TEARS IN TRAUMA RECOVERY WORK

Native peoples of the far north who live in harsh and cold climates have between 180 and 300 words for snow. Compare that to the relatively scant number of words we have for tears—cry, sob, whimper, bawl, snivel, wail, all words that conjure sadness and gloom. In fact, tears are so often associated with sadness that we might assume that when therapists cry it is because something in the interaction with a client has caused them to feel a sense of loss or sadness. But there are many different kinds of tears that are a normal—though far from routine—part of doing therapy with severely damaged trauma survivors. I describe some of these different types of tears in the stories below. If any of these stories bring a tear to your eye then you will understand the experience of therapists who cry.

Tears of Recognition

We listen as a woman remembers her younger self. We can envision the child who was left behind to face terrible circumstances on her own. She paints an image of a child who sits straining to hear her mother's steps as they grow fainter and fainter on the cobblestone driveway. Or the girl who takes one last longing look as the car drives her to the her new foster home and her mother's image grows smaller and smaller in the distance. These visual images of lost and lonely children draw the therapist into the life of the trauma survivor who is not just telling a story, she is sharing a picture of herself. These clearly drawn images of childhood suffering pull tears from even the most objective listener.

Paula's Story

Paula was just a child when her abuse began, maybe six or seven years old. She recalls her mother putting her on the bus to go visit her cousins in South Carolina and she remembers being excited. We can see the little girl with ribbons in her hair and a smile on her face. But her summer in the country was anything but idyllic.

A few days after she arrived, Paula's uncle began taking her behind the tractor in the barn and raping her. When she started to cry, he put his hand over her mouth and called her "a little whore." He then gave her some brown liquid to drink, a liquid that made the pain seem less, but a liquid that began a 30-year history of alcohol abuse.

When she returned home from her "visit," Paula was no longer a naïve child. She was a sullen girl who stayed in her room and dreamt of suicide. When she could no longer endure the feelings of self-loathing, Paula ran to a life on the streets, a life filled with drugs, abuse, and torment.

At this point, the therapist's image of Paula as a distinct and unique hurt child begins to fade and Paula blends into one more abused woman, a woman with a sad story, but no longer the stark visual image that had caused the therapist to well up with tears. One of the great tragedies of abuse is that it robs women and men of their unique identities. Personhood disappears in the quicksand of trauma.

Paula only regains her individuality when the story changes again. Now, Paula is lying on the floor as her abusive boyfriend kicks her in the face and the sirens are wailing because a neighbor has called the police. As Paula is being carried from the apartment, a streetwise cop leans over and whispers, "If you stay with him, you are going to die. That man is going to kill you." And then, once again, the therapist can see the face of the little girl on the bus to South Carolina.

Once in court to testify against her boyfriend, Paula can see tears welling up in the judge's eyes. This judge, who had been on the bench for many years, looked Paula in the eyes and said, "I don't often cry in court, but you have me crying now."

Visual images of suffering can move us to tears, whether we are unbiased judges or seemingly objective therapists.

Tears of Compassion and Sorrow

Sometimes a woman's story, whether told individually or in a group, is so overwhelmingly sad that it literally pulls the tears from the therapist's eyes. Often these are stories in which the abuse is coupled with abandonment and profound loss. It is as if we can hear the gospel song, "Sometimes I feel like a motherless child" wailing in the background and we witness the child who is lost and alone, with no place to rest her head. At this moment, the therapist wants to reach across the room and offer comfort.

Wanda's Story

It was Christmas morning when Wanda heard the loud scream and saw her mother tumble down the stairs, clutching a bottle of whiskey. Even though she was only five years old, Wanda knew what to do: she called the police and waited, sucking her thumb, until the ambulance came to take her mother away. As they were leaving the house, the medic turned to Wanda and said in a rather matter-of-fact way, "Now you watch, girl, because you're going to have to take care of your momma when this happens again."

And thus began Wanda's ten-year ordeal as a "motherless child." She cooked and cleaned, watched over her mother for signs of a seizure, and stayed in the house. She never went to school, or had friends, and only learned of the world by looking out the window and watching soap operas on TV. Wanda was 15 years old, illiterate and frightened, the first time she walked into a school.

As Wanda told her story, the therapist could feel tears running down her own cheeks. In that moment of compassion, the therapist could touch the pain of that lonely little girl. That shared moment could not change the horror of the past, but it could give the adult Wanda a sense that someone cared and that she was no longer all alone.

Kelly's Story

If you asked her, Kelly would tell you that she had four mothers: her birth mother, whom Kelly met for the first time when Kelly was almost 40; her foster mother, who fed her and cared for Kelly during a severe illness that lasted almost six months; her adopted mother, who died suddenly when Kelly was only six, but who she remembers loved her and made her feel special, and her stepmother, who called Kelly names and made her stand in the closet whenever she was "bad."

Before she was six years old, Kelly had two names, one given to her in foster care and a second by her adopted mother. For a long time, she was not sure who she was, nor was she clear about which of these women deserved the name "mother." One child, two names, four mothers, and an early childhood filled with confusion and abandonment.

What therapist would not feel that pain and would not want to wrap Kelly in her arms with gentle tears meant to offer comfort? Yet the therapist cannot pretend to be "mother number five." As much as we might wish it, the therapist can do no more than bear witness to Kelly's sorrow and to acknowledge her painful realization, "How am I to know what love feels like? Love is just a memory to me."

Tanya's Story

And now, just a brief vignette. At the end of a group dealing with abuse and loss, Tanya looked up as if she had seen a ghost, "My mom died a week after I was born and one day I was looking through some family photos and I thought, 'This is great. I'll find a picture of my mother', and then I remembered, I have no idea what my mother looks like."

Tears of Anger and Despair

Tears of anger and despair seem to come from a different place within the therapist than those of compassion and sadness. We don't want to offer comfort; instead we find ourselves wanting to rail at the universe: "How can this have happened?"

In his much-acclaimed folksong, Bob Dylan sings of "Tears of Rage," the tears that spring from a profound sense of betrayal. And while Dylan is referring to betrayal between father and daughter, soldier and country, tears of anger are shed every time we feel that a grave breach of trust has occurred. Anger, however, surprises us. It is not always directed where we might expect. Sometimes we are angry at the world for what it has done to the survivor of trauma and sometimes we are angry, appropriately or not, with the survivor herself.

Kali's Story

At the beginning of group work, all Kali could remember was that she had been afraid since she was six years old. Mostly, she was afraid of all of the beatings. Her mother would beat her when she was late coming home, when she forgot to wash her dishes after a meal, when she was too quiet or too noisy. Her mother would beat Kali when she was in a drunken rage just looking for someone to hit.

When Kali got older, her mother would leave her to babysit her younger brothers and sisters while Mom went out to party. And one day, one of her mother's many boyfriends came over and began slapping Kali for not being polite. But slapping was not all he did. He raped Kali until the pain got so bad that she could do nothing but stare into space.

The next day, Kali wanted to tell her mother what had happened, but she knew her mother would never believe her, so—in an act of amazing courage—she went to school and told her teacher. The teacher was horrified and immediately went to the school counselor who called Child Welfare. The Child Welfare administrators decided that Kali's home was too unsafe so they removed Kali and her siblings and placed them all in foster care. Kali spent the next nine years of her young life moving from one abusive foster home to another.

How can this happen? How can courage be rewarded with punishment? How can a system designed to provide care and protection betray the hopes of a young child?

This time the therapist's tears were tears of despair, and of anger, tears toward a universe that left both Kali and the therapist feeling powerless.

Lila's Story

Women who have been abused and marginalized have clearly lived lives of pain and despair. So what right do therapists have to feel anger and disappointment towards them? But, sometimes we do.

Lila's father, a well-respected lawyer, began raping her when she was ten. In between assaults, he threatened her and told her that no one would ever believe her and that, if she told, she would be sent to a mental hospital with "all the other crazy people."

Lila began running away, spending nights in the woods and drinking with her friends, until the police broke up the party and dragged her back home where the rapes were now coupled with beatings. This pattern went on for years, with the alcohol being replaced by cocaine and then heroin. And during all this time, Lila completed high school, took ballet lessons, and prepared for college.

Despite her amazing resilience, however, Lila's story went the way you might expect. Drugs held an ever-increasing power over her life. She took to the streets, began prostituting to pay for drugs, and eventually was arrested for possession of heroin.

Lila knew that she could not go on this way and when she left jail, she sought therapy. For two years, she participated in both individual and group therapy and began to gain insight into her behavior and trust in the therapists who worked with her. She gave up drugs, went to college for a degree in social work, got her own apartment, began a new relationship, adopted a puppy from the shelter, and, in short, became a poster child for recovery. For seven years, she lived the life she could have had before the abuse started.

And then she began to miss group sessions. The other group members started to worry about her and one of them called the police. Her therapist waited anxiously for news of Lila. Then the police officer who had gone to check on Lila called to report that she had been found dead in her apartment with nothing but a whimpering dog and a needle in her neck.

Lila's story ends tragically and one would expect that the therapist, along with others, would be filled with sadness and compassion. And they were, but mixed in were intense feelings of anger. How could she have betrayed her own success? How could she have let down her fellow group members for whom Lila's recovery was a sign that they, too, could free themselves from the past? And how could she betray those therapists who had worked so hard and cared so much to help her? At her funeral, mourners cried tears of sadness, but they also cried "tears of rage."

Tears of Triumph and Joy

Most often tears are associated with the sad and painful things in life, the hurts and the tragedies. This is especially true for trauma survivors where pain, betrayal, abandonment, and lifelong scarring are part of the pattern. But every so often, something comes along that makes us swell with happiness. It is the feeling we have when we see a child who has "beaten" cancer, or when we watch the victory of a wounded soldier who can compete without his legs. The triumph of the human spirit is powerful and when we see a survivor who has survived and truly flourished, our tears are tears of pure joy and pride. At times we even feel honored to witness such triumph.

Jen's Story

Jen's home life was far from idyllic. Her mother drank, her father was angry, and her older sister prostituted when the family needed extra money, but Jen always felt that, in the midst of instability, her mother loved her and would keep her safe. Jen often slept in her mother's bed, where she felt warm and protected. Then one night, Jen crept out of bed to go the bathroom. When she returned, she found her mother sprawled on the floor, dead from a massive heart attack.

Since there was really no one at home to take care of her, and since her mother was gone, Jen was shipped off to a distant cousin where she became the family maid. She cooked, cleaned, and babysat, but she did not cry.

Her older sister told her that crying was not allowed: "Momma is dead and gone and you will just have to make do."

Unfortunately, for Jen, "making do" meant hitting the streets in search of someone who would love and protect her the way her mother had. Since she was a young, pretty woman, there were plenty of "gentlemen" who were only too glad to take care of her.

Jen spent almost 25 years on the streets, prostituting, dancing in high-end clubs, and taking every drug she was offered. On the streets, Jen was raped, contracted HIV, and was eventually arrested for distributing heroin. Jen felt at the end of her struggle; she was never going to recover that feeling of love that she had before her mother died.

And then Jen had what she calls a vision. She was standing at a fork in the road. To the right was another bag of heroin and drowsy oblivion and to the left were a group of women on their way to a homeless shelter. Jen went left and was welcomed as a "sister in recovery." She was no longer alone; she was with others, as hungry for love as she was.

Jen has been sober for over ten years. She mentors other women and continues to attend group therapy sessions. But it is her triumph over pain and longing that brings tears. In one group, she leaned toward a woman who was struggling with domestic violence; she held out her hand. "I've been where you are now. Just take my hand. I will pull you up. I will pull you up."

There was not a dry eye in the room. Jen was able to share her triumph with the other women and the whole group felt joy for and with her.

Private Tears

Sometimes, although we hate to admit it and may even be told that it is wrong, a woman's words reach out and touch our own experience. In one group, a woman wept as she described how she thought of her mother every single day since her death 23 years ago. The therapist sat back in her chair and felt her eyes well up. "My mother died 15 years ago and I think of her every day, too," she said. A moment of shared remembrance and loss. The therapist was not crying for the woman, but rather they were crying with one another, and in that moment the humanness and connection of all the women in the group were palpable.

In another group, a woman shared her longing for her mother who had died only five months previously. She told of how she still drove by her mother's apartment, hoping that she would see her sitting on the porch. Another woman looked over and asked where the apartment was and what unit the first woman's mother had occupied.

"She was in unit 25."

"Oh my God! Was your mother Jessie Robbins?"

"Did you know my mother?"

"Of course I did." The second woman then took out her phone and said, "Look here. I have a picture of me and your mother sitting on the porch."

The room grew silent and everyone watched as the grieving woman looked at the picture of her mother. Every group member who wished to feel the presence of someone lost sat frozen and then they shared a solemn moment of gentle crying. The women stood, held hands, and experienced their collective humanity.

CONCLUSION AND RECOMMENDATIONS

Stories of trauma and abuse are horrific. Crying is a form of bearing witness to the pain of others.

Our tears as therapists may come when we break through and move past labels and recognize the fullness of the women before us, as we become humans in a room together, witnessing suffering, growth, and recovery. Tears may come to a therapist when witnessing and experiencing the connections in a group, and because the therapist is necessarily and inherently a part of the group, too. And a therapist's tears may be a glimmer of validation to a woman who has rarely experienced empathy to her pain.

There is no way to predict when *your* tears will emerge in doing trauma recovery work, if tears emerge at all. If any of the stories above brought you to tears, perhaps you can pause to reflect on them. Was there something in the tales that resonated? That particularly moved you? Were yours tears of recognition? Tears of sorrow? Tears of anger, or joy? Perhaps these tears are familiar to you in some way. Perhaps they surprised you. In the end, after all, they are your tears and only you will ever know their true meaning.

NOTES

1. In this chapter, I focus on trauma recovery work with women and the stories I tell are based on women who have experienced trauma.
2. Details of each of the cases presented in this chapter have been changed to maintain anonymity.

REFERENCES

Harris, M., & Community Connections Trauma Work Group (1998). *Trauma recovery and empowerment: A clinician's guide for working with women in groups.* New York, NY: The Free Press/Simon & Schuster.

Herman, J. (1992). *Trauma and recovery: The aftermath of violence—from domestic abuse to political terror.* New York, NY: Basic Books/Perseus Books Group.

CHAPTER 10

TEARS AND THE DYING CLIENT[1]

Eleanor F. Counselman

> When the Whites[2] first came to see me they presented an almost classic case for couples treatment. Married for 30 years, they had grown children, all living away from home. Dick was in his early 50s, an affable policeman of Irish background. Mary, also in her 50s, worked part-time as a beautician, and was of Italian descent. Mary had recently discovered that Dick had been having an affair and had given him the choice of therapy or divorce. A psychotherapy that began in this benign manner as straightforward marriage counseling turned into my first experience with a terminally ill client who died of cancer during our work together.

This chapter is about my experience as the Whites' therapist during the last year of Mary's life. It is specifically about my self-disclosure and tears as I helped a couple say goodbye to each other.

PSYCHOTHERAPY AT THE END OF LIFE

To set the stage for discussing psychotherapy at the end of life and its unique emotional implications for the therapist, I begin by reviewing literature on working with terminally ill clients. Specifically, I discuss the relationship between cancer and emotions, individually and within the family, and then discuss aspects of psychotherapy unique to working with cancer patients and patients at the end of their life. While I have focused on cancer here, both because of its prevalence (according to the American Cancer Society, cancer accounts for nearly one of every four deaths in the United States and one in every seven deaths worldwide) and also because cancer is what Mary and her family struggled with, the implications of the emotional impact of cancer and the unique aspects of therapy with cancer patients can be expanded to other medical conditions (though certainly the specifics of any given medical condition have implications for the experience of the individual and family).

Emotions and Cancer

The relationship between cancer and emotions has been studied extensively. On one hand, there is significant research and debate regarding the impact of emotions on the incidence, course, and progression of cancer. On the other hand, there is much to be said about the emotional impact of being diagnosed and living with cancer. It becomes quickly clear how the relationship between cancer and emotions can be conceived of as bidirectional. One meta-analysis found psychological distress, such as depression, anxiety, and poor quality of life, to be associated with an increased risk of getting cancer (prospectively), and cancer mortality and poorer prognosis in those who had already been diagnosed (Chida, Hamer, Wardle, & Steptoe, 2008). In a meta-analysis looking at depression specifically, Pinquart and Duberstein (2010a) found that having a diagnosis of depression and higher levels of depressive symptoms predicted elevated cancer mortality. On the other hand, studies have found an association between positive social networks and better illness trajectory. Pinquart and Duberstein's (2010b) meta-analysis of the association between social networks and cancer mortality found a clear relationship between longevity of cancer patients and their perception of social support. While research on the relationship between cancer and emotions is nuanced and complex, I make note of these studies to highlight the strong association between psychological distress/well-being and course of illness. It appears that greater psychological distress is related to a poorer prognosis while greater well-being, particularly in the form of perceived social support, is related to better prognosis.

While social support is clearly important in the quality of life of cancer patients, it can be challenging for those most closely involved, particularly family members, who are themselves affected by the cancer diagnosis. Indeed, one member's cancer impacts the whole family. Meissner (1993) observed that, while some families emotionally decompensate, others react by functioning at more adaptive and mature levels than before the illness. K. Wilber (1988) wrote about the role of the support person as both "painful and profoundly redeeming" (p. 141). Kübler-Ross (1969) wrote, "we cannot help the terminally ill patient in a really meaningful way if we do not include his family" (p. 157).

In looking at the relationship between cancer and emotions, both intra- and interindividually, we must take note that, on some level, we are describing a relationship between the mind and the body: how emotions affect our physical body and how the physical body (in this case, cancer within the body) affects our emotional state. This is a discussion pertinent to the subject of this chapter—tears—which are a physical manifestation of our emotional state, a parallel of the mind–body connection that is so often discussed in working with cancer.

Therapy With Cancer Patients

Studies that look at the effectiveness of therapy with cancer patients often cite improved quality of life and/or reduced emotional distress, depression, anxiety, or even pain. Some researchers have demonstrated that psychotherapy not only improves quality of life but extends it as well (e.g., Spiegel, Bloom, Kraemer, & Gottheil, 1989; Fawzy, Canada, & Fawzy, 2003). Spiegel et al.'s (1989) landmark study on this topic looked at women with metastasized breast cancer and demonstrated a powerful link between participating in support-expressive group psychotherapy and longer survival. Fawzy, Canada, and Fawzy (2003) found that group cognitive-behavioral therapy was associated with a decreased risk of death. Other studies are less clear about the relationship between mortality and psychotherapy (Coyne, Stefanek, & Palmer, 2007), though the role of psychotherapy in helping with a greater sense of well-being and reduced psychological distress is widely accepted within the psycho-oncological community.

How does a client's cancer affect psychotherapy? Adams-Silvan (1994) wrote about her psychoanalytic psychotherapy with a woman dying of cancer. The time pressure she felt made it impossible to be neutral about subject matter. Instead, she actively encouraged her patient to express any and all feelings, without regard to the therapist's feelings. Such expression might be difficult or impossible with people in her life toward whom she needed to be protective (family, friends, etc.). She also helped her patient resolve burdens from the past, thus freeing her to engage more in the present. Although her patient had generally oedipal concerns, she felt that the technical decisions she made were more like those she would make with preoedipal patients. The illness-created psychological regression may create more primitive demands on the therapist than would otherwise occur. Indeed, Meissner (1993), in describing the tremendous psychological impact on patients of a cancer diagnosis, noted that the diagnosis often provokes extreme mobilization of primitive defenses.

Both Adams-Silvan (1994) and Cole (1992) noted that therapy with a dying client inevitably feels different to the therapist and requires technical modifications. Adams-Silvan felt a "relaxation from a long personal and professional accumulation of technical guidelines, experience, requirements, and even strictures" (p. 339). Cole wrote of changes in the frame that allow the therapist to be more accessible and real, thus reducing client anxiety and fears of object loss, but also can emotionally drain the therapist and distract from transferential and interpretive work.

Richman (1995) noted the danger of terminal despair and the role a psychotherapist can play in preventing it. Such psychotherapy is inevitably a profound experience for the therapist as well. He concluded that an important goal of psychotherapy with a terminally ill patient should be to help the person die in a state of psychological well-being. Richman emphasized the awareness of countertransference (both positive and negative). Confrontation of one's own attitudes about illness and death is essential. The core of such therapy must be one human being relating to another.

Bartley (2012), in outlining a mindfulness-based cognitive therapy approach to working with cancer patients, described three specific challenges that the therapist may confront in working with cancer patients. First, she noted that working with death and dying inevitably brings up the therapist's own anxieties around mortality. Second, she described how working with cancer patients brings up the practitioner's attitudes and feelings about hospitals, medical interventions (needles, blood, chemotherapy, surgery) and other related issues such as hair loss, stoma bags, nausea, and pain. Third, she discussed the ways in which therapists can begin to experience their own health anxieties or hypervigilance about somatic concerns. She stressed that this is not uncommon given that even a person in seemingly perfect health can get cancer and therefore therapists working with cancer patients are reminded time and again of their own vulnerability.

MacCormack et al. (2001) conducted a qualitative study to examine cancer patients' experience of psychotherapy at the end of life and found three factors that patients reported to be most beneficial. First, patients focused on the relational experience as the most helpful aspect of therapy (as opposed to specific techniques). Second, therapy provided a unique, safe space for patients to explore thoughts and feelings they may not have felt comfortable sharing with others. Third, the therapist was seen as an experienced professional who truly cared: "connecting with their therapists as people and not just professionals meant patients could experience them as helpful because, in the end, they were able to show they 'cared'" (p. 59). The qualities that patients emphasized as being most important in their therapists were that they were easy to be with, safe, genuine, warm, understanding, and, "above all, truly cared" (p. 59).

Through this brief review of literature relevant to the topic of psychotherapy at the end of life, we can see that there is an inherent emotional impact on the therapist of working with a person who is dying, and his or her family. Therapists must be willing to enter into a human relationship with their client who is facing one of life's most difficult existential challenges. It is not hard to imagine how therapist's emotional reactions, self-disclosure, and tears become a relevant topic to working with the dying client.

THERAPISTS' TEARS IN THERAPY WITH THE DYING CLIENT

The first six months of treatment with the Whites was standard couples counseling. They worked hard to understand Dick's affair, began to communicate in new, more intimate ways, and started to have fun with each other. At Mary's request, Dick began to plan "dates" for them. Mary was able to let go of some old anger about being left at home with young children. She had been treated for breast cancer a few years earlier but had been given a good prognosis. In therapy we talked about her long-buried resentment that her husband had not been supportive during her treatment; for example, he would get irate if the radiation treatment was late and he was kept waiting. They talked about that experience and both realized that his withdrawal had been self-protective. Although Dick was uncomfortable with direct expression of feelings, he clearly loved his wife and family. The music was there even if the words were not. I left for vacation in August expecting to discuss termination when I returned.

Our first session in September brought the first of many pieces of bad news: Mary had experienced a recurrence of her breast cancer. The cancer had spread to her spine, and she was undergoing tests to determine the extent of the metastasis. I was shocked and speechless; I felt tears come to my eyes. The Whites did not comment on my tears but detailed the medical plans. This time Dick was involved, attending every doctor's appointment. They did not seem to be as filled with doom as I felt. In retrospect, I think my oncology knowledge at that moment was probably greater. Or perhaps they were still in shock.

Although I had 25 years of experience as a therapist, my first reaction to Mary's illness was that I did not know what to do. (In retrospect, I see this as both a professional and an existential reaction; none of us really knows what to do in the face of death.) I thought perhaps I should refer the Whites to a therapist more expert in handling serious illness. Perhaps I also longed to escape the pain I knew was ahead. My mother had died a hard death from cancer seven years earlier, and I did not look forward to revisiting that experience. Ultimately I decided that the Whites would experience a referral as rejection and abandonment. I decided that the connection the Whites and I had made was more important than another therapist's greater experience with serious illness and that I would get consultation for myself as needed.

I believe that this decision to place priority on the connection was correct and laid the foundation for the rest of the Whites' treatment. To work with death, one must be alive and present in the room. Experience and training are much less important than the capacity to *be there*. In addition, it is inevitable that certain modifications in the frame will occur. This topic has been well described by Cole (1992). Such modifications might include changes in therapy appointments due to medical needs, changes in location (e.g., home or hospital visits), adding family members for family sessions, and greater self-disclosure or transparency on the part of the therapist.

I am fortunate to be a member of a long-term peer consultation group. I brought up the Whites at our next meeting and asked for advice. My group encouraged me to share some of my feelings with the Whites, perhaps even my own personal experience with my mother's cancer. I reflected on my fear of crying and realized that I was afraid of not being able to stop crying if I started—a fear clients have often expressed to me. I decided my first priority was to be present with the Whites, whatever that might bring up for me.

At our next meeting, the Whites had the results of the tests: Mary's original cancer, a particularly aggressive type, had metastasized but not very far. Radiation, then powerful chemotherapy, was planned. I asked the Whites about our work. They said they wanted a place to talk to each other about their feelings (and, I thought to myself, to say goodbye to each other). The Whites also asked me to help them talk to their children about the cancer. I decided to tell them that I had lost my mother to cancer, a less treatable kind, and that Mary's cancer touched me very much. I told them that my mother had not been able to talk with me or our family about her illness, and I found that a great loss. I suggested that at some point they might like to invite the boys in for a family meeting, and they thought that would be a good idea.

Mary's radiation was tiring but not terrible. Dick was able to take her to most appointments and did not "blow up" when Radiology was running late. The next phase, chemotherapy, was much worse. Mary lost her hair almost immediately, evoking sad memories for me. Although Dick denied it, Mary felt unattractive to her husband and would not allow him to see her bald. She became constantly nauseated, and in sympathy my stomach became upset during our meetings (and would immediately calm down after the Whites left). Dick remained steadfast, gradually assuming more of the cooking and household chores.

In January more tests were run; and I dreaded the results. Dick began our meeting by saying, "The chemo didn't work." Mary and I both started to cry, and Dick handed each of us a tissue. (It was a matter of personal pride at the time with him to remain dry-eyed.) I leaned forward and said, "I am so sorry." We sat quietly together for a few minutes, terribly sad. My tears felt natural and were for Mary, not my mother. We then talked about the latest treatment recommendations and about the family. The Whites decided it was time for a family meeting.

The family meeting, held in February, was framed as a chance for everyone to talk together about Mary's cancer. The Whites were a family who didn't "do feelings." The eldest son, Todd, began the meeting by aggressively (the best defense is a good offense) asking his mother for the facts of her situation. The conversation soon moved to the role of feelings in their family and to the fact that none of the children had ever seen their father cry. I said that cancer seemed like something people might cry about. Mary grieved that she would not live to see grandchildren, and the children looked helpless in the face of her tears. The middle son, Brian, said that seeing his mother weep made him uncomfortable and he wished he knew what to do. Mary said that what she wanted was to be allowed to have her feelings without their withdrawing. The session ended movingly, with each child giving her a long hug.

During the spring Mary held her own. She continued medical treatments that left her tired and sick. Dick was attentive and patient. I wondered how he stood it, because Mary often made him the brunt of her rage about her situation (see Wilber (1988) for a thorough discussion of the role of the cancer support person). I pointed out that cancer was the uninvited, unwelcome intruder in their lives and that Mary's rage was about that. Dick told more of his story, including the painful loss of his mother. As a couple, they completed painful but necessary tasks, such as signing wills and choosing a cemetery plot. Dick's Irish humor carried us all through the cemetery selection with such quips as, "She didn't like the Arlington plot . . . too noisy . . . might keep her awake at night."

During this period I saw my role as helping them have an ongoing conversation about the unbearable. I took to bringing snacks to my office to eat after they left because I felt so depleted after sessions. I arranged consultation for myself with a therapist who specialized in treatment of patients with medical illness to make sure I was on the right track with the Whites and (more importantly) to feel less alone in the work. I read Pollin's (1995) *Medical Crisis Counseling*.

By summertime, Mary needed a lot of medication for pain. It became very difficult for her to negotiate the stairs to my office. I was touched by Dick's tenderness as he held his wife's arm to help her walk. They looked like an elderly couple. The contrast between Mary's condition and my own good health—two women close in age—was a reminder of the randomness of life. Wilber (1988) notes that illness inevitably raises the question, "Why me?" I found myself thinking, "Why not me?" I left for my vacation thinking about home visits. When I returned, Dick called to say Mary could no longer manage my stairs, and we decided that I would come to their home for the next visit. However, on the morning of the visit, Dick called to say that Mary was in the hospital. He asked if I would lead a family session in her hospital room, and I agreed.

The meeting had an upsetting start. When I walked into Mary's hospital room, I saw an old woman curled up in bed and quickly apologized for being in the wrong room. Mary assured me it was her. I was stunned by the devastation of her illness. Mary's parents attended the family meeting as well as Dick and her sons. Everyone was very distressed and found it hard to talk. In addition, the constant intrusions of hospital life were distracting. However, an important question was asked and answered: how did Mary wish to live out her remaining days? She said that she wanted as much time with her family as possible; only that was important to her. On the way out, Todd asked me if I did a lot of family meetings in the hospital. I answered truthfully, saying this was my first one. He did not say anything, but later in the fall he came for several individual sessions to talk about his mother's death. I believe he appreciated my honesty.

The family gave her what she wanted. A hospital bed was set up at home in the dining room so she could always be near people. She had good home care and was relatively pain-free. Her parents moved in to help, and her children moved home. I continued to see Dick every few weeks as support. Mary lived for two months after that family meeting and died with her husband holding her hand.

Before Mary's death I asked Dick if I could come to the wake. I was raised in a culture which did not use the term "wake"; instead we called it "paying your respects." I wanted to pay my respects to the hard work of this family. The wake was significant in two ways: first, I had never seen a client of mine laid out in a casket. She looked peaceful but so different from her old self. Second, I briefly entered the Whites' regular life and saw them with their friends and family. As therapists, we rarely participate in our clients' "real worlds."

Dick came to see me a few more times to grieve, and to my surprise the children asked for a final family meeting. The holidays were approaching and no one knew how to have Christmas without their mother. Once again I framed our task as talking about what people were feeling. They talked about how sad they were and reminisced about past holidays with their mother. Everyone feared that without her the family would not stay together. I reminded them that each of them had a role in deciding whether the family remained close. We also spoke of their mother living on in their memories and the stories they will tell their future children. We agreed that our work together was over and said goodbye.

CONCLUSION AND RECOMMENDATIONS

I will always remember the Whites. They grew as a family in the midst of their pain, and I was happy to have been part of it. I believe that they connected to me as well as they did because I decided to be open and real with them, which encouraged them to be open and real with each other. I learned not to fear crying with a client. I had the opportunity to see a family talk about illness and death as my own family could not, and that was healing for me in the way our work as therapists often is.

My recommendations to therapists treating seriously ill or dying clients, with specific regard for the topic of tears in therapy, are:

1. Be as present in the work as you can be. Consider greater self-disclosure, including emotional self-disclosure, than usual if it will enhance the connection.
2. Be prepared for your own strong reactions, for example, tears or somatic disturbances. Strong emotions are sometimes experienced most powerfully in the body. Working with terminally ill patients can stir up very difficult feelings, and a focus on bodily sensation can be a window into affect that the mind can't quite tolerate.
3. Be clear about the task of therapy. You may be tempted to problem solve to avoid helpless feelings. Your work is to help your client bear the unbearable. This means bearing the unbearable yourself.

4. Be prepared for frame modifications and be flexible but thoughtful about their meanings.
5. Do not do this type of therapy alone; it is too demanding. Outside consultation offers invaluable perspective and support.
6. Remember that research on patients' experience of psychotherapy at the end of life finds that patients prefer a therapist who can balance professionalism with a personal relationship: patients report it is most "helpful to see someone who [is more] 'objective' [than] family or friends might be . . . Nevertheless participants highlight . . . how important it [is] to engage with someone who [can] connect or relate with them on a personal level" (MacCormack et al., 2001, p. 59). Striking this balance between professionalism, appropriateness, honesty, authenticity, and connection is a—perhaps the most—crucial task in this challenging and fulfilling work.

Although painful and stressful, helping individuals and families manage serious or terminal illness is very rewarding therapy. Therapists can be of tremendous service to individuals and families facing terminal illness, but they must be prepared to have powerful reactions themselves. Therapist tears, reflecting greater emotional self-disclosure than might be appropriate in some other clinical settings, are natural and appropriate for this work.

NOTES

1. Portions of this chapter have been adapted from an article by Eleanor F. Counselman printed in the journal *Psychotherapy*: Copyright © 1997 by the Division of Psychotherapy (29), American Psychological Association. Adapted with permission. The official citation that should be used in referencing original material is: Counselman, E. F. (1997) Self-disclosure, tears and the dying client, *Psychotherapy, 34*(3), 233–237. The use of this information does not imply endorsement by the publisher.
2. Certain biographical information has been changed to protect the identity of the "Whites."

REFERENCES

Adams-Silvan, A. (1994). "That darkness—is about to pass": The treatment of a dying patient. *Psychoanalytic Study of the Child, 49*, 328–348.
American Cancer Society. (2015). *Cancer facts and figures*. Retrieved from http://www.cancer.org/acs/groups/content/@editorial/documents/document/acspc-044552.pdf (accessed November 20, 2016).

Bartley, T. (2012). *Mindfulness-based cognitive therapy for cancer: Gently turning towards*. Chichester, UK: Wiley-Blackwell.

Chida, Y., Hamer, M., Wardle, J., & Steptoe, A. (2008). Do stress-related psychosocial factors contribute to cancer incidence and survival? A systematic quantitative review of 40 years of inquiry. *National Clinical Practice Oncology, 5*, 466–475.

Cole, A. B. (1992). Frame modifications with a dying client. *Smith College Studies in Social Work, 63*, 313–324.

Counselman, E. F. (1997). Self-disclosure, tears and the dying client. *Psychotherapy, 34*(3), 233–237.

Coyne, J. C., Stefanek, M., & Palmer, S. C. (2007). Psychotherapy and survival in cancer: The conflict between hope and evidence. *Psychological Bulletin, 133*(3), 367.

Fawzy, F. I., Canada, A. L., & Fawzy, N. W. (2003). Malignant melanoma: Effects of a brief, structured psychiatric intervention on survival and recurrence at 10-year follow-up. *Archives of General Psychiatry, 60*, 100–103.

Kübler-Ross, E. (1969). *On death and dying*. New York, NY: Macmillan.

MacCormack, T., Simonian, J., Lim, J., Remond, L., Roets, D., Dunn, S., & Butow, P. (2001). 'Someone who cares': A qualitative investigation of cancer patients' experiences of psychotherapy. *Psycho-Oncology, 10*(1), 52–65.

Meissner, W. W. (1993). The family and cancer. *Psychiatric Annals, 23*(9), 513–518.

Pinquart, M., & Duberstein, P. R. (2010a). Depression and cancer mortality: A meta-analysis. *Psychological Medicine, 40*(11), 1797–1810.

Pinquart, M., & Duberstein, P. R. (2010b). Associations of social networks with cancer mortality: A meta-analysis. *Critical Reviews in Oncology/Hematology, 75*(2), 122–137.

Pollin, I. (1995). *Medical crisis counseling*. New York, NY: W.W. Norton.

Richman, J. (1995). From despair to integrity: An Eriksonian approach to psychotherapy for the terminally ill. *Psychotherapy, 32*(2), 317–322.

Spiegel, D., Bloom, J. R., Kraemer, H. C., & Gottheil, E. (1989). Effect of psychosocial treatment on survival of patients with metastatic breast cancer. *Lancet, 2*, 888–891.

Wilber, K. (1988). On being a support person. *Journal of Transpersonal Psychology, 20*(2), 141–159.

CHAPTER 11

ENTERING THE NO-CRY ZONE: MEN AND THE CHORDS OF CONNECTION

Fredric E. Rabinowitz

> *Zack stared at me. It would be hard not to take note of my watery eyes. He commented, devoid of emotion, "Sorry for making such a big deal out it. It's been 23 years. I've moved on." It was as if he was letting me know that he had violated the male no-cry zone by sharing his sadness and he was apologizing that it had impacted me. I understood that he was operating on the assumption of the "boy code," which warns men that they will be ostracized from the group if they share vulnerable emotions (Rabinowitz & Cochran, 1994). I also knew that this was an opportunity to challenge some of the learned traditional male gender role norms ingrained in Zack, and that doing so might allow him to let go of some of the pain he was holding inside.*

In this chapter, I will discuss some of the basic tenets of therapy with men as they relate to the topic of tears in therapy. I will then present a case to examine the unique challenges, as well as opportunities for growth, that can accompany therapists' tears with male clients.

THERAPY WITH MEN

Men often resist coming to therapy even when they know they need help. When a man comes in for a consultation, the situation tends to be relatively extreme. Typical ways of coping are not working. While the presentation of an issue may be described in a calm manner, underneath there is often fear, anxiety, and shame (Shepard & Rabinowitz, 2013). The shame of feeling like one has "not taken care of his business" can overshadow the issue that precipitated his predicament. Most therapists are used to their female clients sharing strong emotion, but are often unprepared for the powerful emotions of a man. Having been socialized to be calm and stoic in the face of adversity, many men can tell a story of hardship, pain, and suffering without shedding a tear. In fact, as a society we have gotten used to this type of presentation and think of it as normal.

For therapy to be effective with men, it is important to allow a male client to tell his own story his own way (Rabinowitz & Cochran, 2002). This often means that the therapist must be patient and listen for the subtle and important themes that arise organically from the way a man describes his life. While men experience strong emotion, they have been trained from childhood to avoid putting these emotions into words. To express pain, shock, sadness, or fear is a threat to the unwritten rules of masculinity that keep these reactions hidden (Rabinowitz & Cochran, 1994). Instead, boys are taught to override their painful and fearful emotional states, using humor, toughness, or stoicism as a response. This leads to a very limited repertoire in terms of emotional expression. In contrast to the way women are socialized, boys and men have few words to describe their inner experience.

One of the major roles a therapist plays in working with men is to help with emotional expression. This does not mean purely filling in the emotional word as the man describes his experience, but rather utilizing the experience itself as a portal to emotional depth (Rabinowitz & Cochran, 2002). This means listening to his vocabulary, his action words, and his external perceptions as ways to intervene. By utilizing metaphors and analogies, a man more readily connects to his emotions, labeled in a way that fits with his experience of the world (McKelley, 2014). For instance, to a man who grew up in a military family that moved frequently and who tells a painful story about divorce in a detached way, a therapist might respond with action words (to bring energy and emotion into the room) that utilize the man's own metaphors for life: "It sounds like you were well practiced for leaving from all the moving you did, but you weren't really prepared to be left." Ultimately, a man in therapy finds his own way of tapping into his internal landscape and the job of the therapist is to facilitate that with understanding, compassion, and genuine interest.

TEARS IN THERAPY WITH MEN

When Zack[1] came to treatment, I did not initially believe that we would engage on a deep emotional level. I saw his muscular body type, the baseball cap he wore and, combined with my prior knowledge that he worked in law enforcement, I assumed he would have trouble accessing his emotions. Zack was 35 years old and recently divorced, with a 13-year-old daughter who was living with his ex-wife. Zack's separation and divorce had spanned two years and the loss was still very present for him. He was living in a small apartment only seven blocks from the house where his wife and daughter lived. He consumed himself with his work at the sheriff's department. Despite the traditional masculine values inherent in the police work, he had a gentle demeanor when he spoke. In addition to being an officer, he was a musician who played guitar in an "Indie" rock band. Zack's face became animated as he told me about this hobby and some of his music idols like Bob Dylan, Bruce Springsteen, and Jackson Browne.

At first glance, Zack's situation seemed pretty typical for a recently divorced guy. He was feeling the loss of family and meaning in his life. While his job kept him busy, it also consumed his emotional energy, leaving him with little chance to unwind. Music was a primary outlet for Zack, and it became clear that playing his guitar was a sort of lifeline for him when things got bleak. However, recently he had been having trouble getting motivated to play. In fact, he had even been struggling to find his appetite, and his sleep was sketchy at best. Zack ruminated about how everything had fallen apart since the divorce. Our initial sessions focused on his current functioning with brief forays into the past, mainly about how he and his wife had gotten to the point of calling it quits. To use a metaphor consistent with Zack's interests: listening to him in these early sessions was like listening to the words of a song, but the melody was not yet audible; while Zack was open with the facts, he was hesitant to share his deeper emotions. I had the sense that the work we were doing was an overture to a larger composition that was not yet clear to me, that something loud and intense was waiting beneath this more cautious prelude. I didn't want to rush Zack, respecting his own tempo, but I anticipated that, at some point, the key would change. In the meantime, as I expected, having weekly meetings to simply process what was going on his life led to improvement in his mood and self-care. He reported being more energized and less ruminative. He told me he looked forward to our sessions. He started to pick up his guitar more and more, and would sometimes talk about music at great length, quoting song lyrics and referencing musical legends. Zack enjoyed sharing his passion.

It was not until our eighth session that the key changed. He had started our meeting by saying he wasn't sure what he should talk about. Everything was going OK on the surface, but something felt a little off.

"There is something deeper there I just can't put my finger on," he said. In order to help him put words to the feeling, I asked him if there was a song that might reflect his mood. With another man, I might have asked him to describe what it felt like in his body, but given Zack's musical passion, this felt most congruent. Without hesitation, Zack said, "It's like something that would play at the beginning of a horror film. You know, building in tension, dissonant, minor key. Something to put you on the edge of your seat." He paused, and then added, "The type of music that makes you feel uneasy in your stomach," making the connection to the feeling in his body himself.

"Is that how you feel now?" I asked. Zack nodded. "When did this come on?"

Zack explained that he had dropped off his daughter at his ex-wife's house, and that she had needed help bringing her suitcase and schoolbooks inside, so he went with her. "I looked around at what used to be my house. I felt like I was going to throw up."

"What was it about the house that brought this on?" I asked.

"I don't know," Zack paused, but then he pressed on. "It felt claustrophobic. Things were messy and cluttered. There were dust balls. I guess I hadn't gone inside for a while, because it took me by surprise. When I lived there everything was in its place. The furniture was orderly. I cleaned every couple of days. Something felt wrong today . . . ominous. Like that horror-movie music." I asked Zack if he had ever had this feeling before. He sat back in his chair and gazed to his left as if he was recalling an event from his past. Silence filled the room as he seemed to access a memory.

"This is weird," Zack finally said, his voice low. "I'm remembering the house I grew up in. Something about walking into Tina's place with it so out of order, it reminded me of my childhood home."

"What do you mean?"

"I'm not sure I can talk about it." Suddenly, his eyes started to get moist. I was taken back a bit, but felt a surge of my own emotions, especially sadness.

"Did something happen at your house, Zack?" I asked, but Zack couldn't speak. A tear rolled down his cheek. For me, everything in the room faded away except for Zack's face. For a moment, it was like hearing music without words.

After about two minutes, with an unfocused glaze, he began, "I was 12 years old when I came home from school one day. Mom used to always be in the house when I got in. She would make me some food and we would talk. It was a part of my everyday ritual. But on that day, she was nowhere to be seen. The house looked out of order. There was a vacuum cleaner out in the middle of the living room. The couch was at a weird angle. I called out to her and got no response. Something was wrong. I could tell." At this point, Zack started to hyperventilate a bit and his cadence quickened. "I went to the upstairs bathroom and saw her lying on the floor, sprawled out. I ran over and said 'Mom, Mom.' No response. There was some blood. I screamed louder, 'Mom! Mom!'" Zack looked terrified and he started to weep uncontrollably.

Immediately, my own eyes watered. I sensed the pain he felt as a child—the surprise and the helplessness. Rarely do I cry in sessions, but this caught me off guard. Emotionally, I felt his vulnerability: surprised by his raw emotion, lost in the moment, not knowing how to soothe him. His intense reaction seemed to touch on every abandonment scene I had ever gone through or witnessed in my personal life and in my life as a therapist. But as fast as the emotion had come to Zack, it left like a passing thunderstorm, a quick crescendo fading to mute. I sensed there was a lot more pain, but this is what he could share with me now. Walking into his ex-wife's house was the trigger, but he had delayed fully responding until he was in the safe confines of my office. I wondered what else was fueling the tears. Zack apologized for being so emotional and then, in a rather matter of fact way, told me that his mom had suffered a heart attack that day and had passed away. "My life changed," he said, and then he looked directly up at me.

It would be hard not to take note of my watery eyes. He commented, devoid of emotion, "Sorry for making such a big deal out it. It's been 23 years. I've moved on." It was as if he was letting me know that he had violated the male no-cry zone by sharing his sadness and he was apologizing that it had impacted me. I understood that he was operating on the assumption of the "boy code," which warns men that they will be ostracized from the group if they share vulnerable emotions (Rabinowitz & Cochran, 1994). I also knew that this was an opportunity to challenge some of the learned traditional male gender role norms, and that doing so might allow him to let go of some of the pain he was holding inside.

"It's OK to express yourself, Zack. I am not at all bummed about it," I said, trying to use language that would bridge the gap between the "boy code" we both knew, and the deeper emotional world we had just accessed. I ventured a metaphor I thought might resonate with him: "It's okay to let the music come. This is a place where it is safe to cry, laugh, or whatever."

"That wasn't a laugh, Fred," he responded. "I don't like telling that story because it tends to have that effect on people."

"You mean the tear thing?"

"Yes. It taps something deep in people. I try not to talk about it. You okay, Fred?"

The tables were turned here. Zack felt like he had done some damage to me: he had caused a fellow man to cry. "What do you mean, Zack?"

"I made you cry. If I was at work, and someone told me a sad story, I don't think it would be good for them to see a cop cry."

"That's interesting," I continued. "How is it for you to see me cry, the professional therapist?"

"Honestly, it's very weird. I can't remember seeing any of my guy friends cry, ever. Never saw my dad cry at all. Even with my mom dying on him, he trucked on."

"So when you cried here, it wasn't OK for you?" I asked.

"Privately I can cry. No one sees my weakness," he replied. "So as long as it is private, it's okay."

"Do you think I am weak for showing my tears, too?" I asked, curious about what he was going to project on to me.

"I see you as sensitive. That can be a weakness or a strength, I guess."

"Is that how you feel about your own tears?" I probed.

"I don't know. When I get into this mood, I usually pull out my guitar and play. In fact, that is when I am the most soulful in my playing. Sometimes I write some lyrics, mess with chords, and then come up with some music that kind of matches my sadness."

"Too bad I don't have a guitar handy," I responded, trying to really understand his process with this very difficult emotion for many men. "How did your dad end up dealing with the loss of your mom?"

"Hah. I wish I knew. I felt like he became more stern and less communicative. I just took on some of the chores my mom did, like cleaning the house. I learned to make my own food and cook for him. We would sit in front of the television when he got home and watch sports mainly. That's the only place I saw him get emotional. He cheered for his teams and got mad when things didn't go well."

"What was that like for you?" I asked.

"I laid low. I kept things to myself. I tried to please him and not make life hard. He was a motorcycle cop so I think he just needed a space where he could chill. We never really talked about mom. As I say it, it sounds weird, given she was the main person in both of our lives. I ended up attaching myself to girls after that. Not sure what he did."

"So the girlfriends helped you feel less lonely?"

"You could say that, but they were mainly short-term fixes. Usually I played the role of listener to their stories. I didn't share much of my own.

I learned quickly that when I was open about what happened with my mom, it changed everything. People didn't know what to do or say. I think it overwhelmed them."

"So when you saw me tear up, you shut down because you thought it might mess up the relationship we established."

"I guess that is true."

"Check it out," I replied, knowing that we were in important territory. Here was a chance for us to improvise. "Have you noticed me pulling away or acting strange around you?"

Zack got quiet. "Actually, it has felt pretty good. No one has really stayed connected with me when I have been in this space. You sure you are okay?" he repeated.

I smiled. This was the beginning of our deeper therapeutic work. When Zack came in after this session he allowed himself to "get into that space" and be more open with his emotions in our sessions. It was as if his "life song" could emerge, the melody and lyrics more connected, vibrant, and strong.

CONCLUSION AND RECOMMENDATIONS

When Zack shared his story about finding his mother dead, it was the turning point in our therapy, the emergence of the theme that helped us understand so many other aspects of Zack's world. He trusted me enough to share his honest reaction to walking into his old house. While Zack was genuinely surprised by my tears, my acceptance of him, and also of myself for shedding tears, was a new experience for him, a new refrain. It gave us both a way to talk about the deeper emotions he felt. By exposing the prohibitions on emotional expression learned from his father, Zack was able to confront an element of his internalized male socialization. An intellectual discussion of gender roles would not have made this kind of impact. The learning moment allowed him to test the waters of trust with me. My own vulnerability seemed to give him permission to be real with himself. Our therapy stayed on a deeper level as we explored not only the pain of losing his mother, but also the deprivation he experienced in growing up with an emotionally closed-off father. We also began to understand the disintegration of his marriage in a new way. His fear of sharing deeper emotion had an impact on the limited intimacy he and his wife experienced. Zack realized that he had chosen a woman who would remain distant with him, ultimately disappointing them both. The tears we shared that day provided an opening for Zack and me to challenge his ideas around emotional intimacy.

While not all men who come to therapy shed tears, those who do need to be supported in a way that reduces their shame. I recall one male client who was in therapy to discuss leaving his job and pursuing a new direction. In the first session, I asked if he had the support of his partner. He said "yes," but something in the way he said it pushed me to probe deeper. By inquiring about their relationship, he alluded to something about her health. I followed up and soon he was crying about nearly losing her. I was aware that, with his socialization and with this being his first session of counseling ever, he might feel overwhelmed. I tried to normalize the shedding of tears, but it was too much. He did not return for a second session. He was not psychologically prepared for the intensity. This example suggests that therapists should be careful in eliciting emotion too early from male clients, especially those with a more traditional gender role orientation. Shame around violating the "boy code," even as adult men, is not easily alleviated.

When men do cry in therapy, and as a therapist you find yourself with tears in your own eyes, it is a crucial moment for both participants. While it might be tempting to skip past your own tears to focus on the client, this could be a mistake. For a male client, tears are often taboo. Seeing the tears reflected in his therapist may intensify his shame for shedding them in the first place. To a traditional male, it may be more acceptable for a female therapist to tear up because of our socialization that women tend to be emotional. On the other hand, when a male therapist cries, it may be more conflictual. Indeed, researchers have shown that men tend to have more negative views of their own sex's tears than of females' tears (Lombardo, Cretser, Lombardo, & Mathis, 1983). By breaking the male norms, a man may feel embarrassed and see the male therapist as weak. But if the therapeutic alliance has been built patiently by allowing the client to go at his own pace, it can be a breakthrough moment of emotional release and a reconsideration of the male taboo of expressing sadness through tears.

As a male therapist, it has taken me years to get comfortable with my own large repertoire of emotion. Like many men, I was raised not to show weakness and certainly not to cry. As I have worked through my emotional pain in my own therapy over the years, I have given myself more permission to feel what comes, knowing I have choices about when, where, and how I will express those feelings. It is important that the consulting room be a place where my male clients can express themselves without shame. Shedding tears, and discussing the implications and reactions to those tears, has the potential to be a powerful clinical moment that can reduce stigma and facilitate self-acceptance. It is an intimate expression that can enhance the therapeutic connection and lead to deeper and more productive therapy. Like my tears with Zack, a therapist's tears with another man may lead to improvisation of the ingrained emotional composition, perhaps allowing for new lyrics, new chords, and new connection to begin.

NOTE

1. Details of Zack's (pseudonym) case have been changed to maintain confidentiality.

REFERENCES

Lombardo, W. K., Cretser, G. A., Lombardo, B., & Mathis, S. (1983). Fer cryin' out loud—There is a sex difference. *Sex Roles: A Journal of Research*, 9, 987–995.

McKelley, R. (2014). Pushing haystacks and cracking steel balls: Using metaphors with men. In A. Rochlen and F. E. Rabinowitz (Eds.) *Breaking barriers in counseling men: Insights and innovations* (pp. 9–19). New York, NY: Routledge.

Rabinowitz, F. E., & Cochran, S. V. (1994). *Man alive: A primer of men's issues*. Monterey, CA: Brooks Cole.

Rabinowitz, F. E., & Cochran, S. V. (2002). *Deepening psychotherapy with men*. Washington, DC: American Psychological Association.

Shepard, D., & Rabinowitz, F. E. (2013). The power of shame in depressed men: Implications for counselors. *Journal of Counseling and Development*, 91, 451–457.

CHAPTER 12

M. NIGHT SHYAMALAN'S *THE SIXTH SENSE:* RELATIONAL AUTHENTICITY, SELF-DISCLOSURE, AND A CHILD THERAPIST'S TEARS[1]

Jerrold R. Brandell

> As the scene unfolds, child psychotherapist, Dr. Malcolm Crowe (Bruce Willis), and his latency-aged patient, Cole Sear (Haley Joel Osment), are seated in what appears to be an office.
>
> "I can't be your doctor any more," Dr. Crowe says to his young patient. His voice is strained as he attempts to appear steadfast in his decision. "I'm going to transfer you—"
>
> "Don't fail me," Cole whispers, interrupting him. "You're the only one who can help me."
>
> "I can't help you," Dr. Crowe states, glancing away from his young patient as his eyes fill with tears. Dr. Crowe looks at Cole, who begins to cry, but then quickly averts his gaze again, as he tries to blink the tears from his own eyes.

The case I will discuss in this chapter on therapist's tears in psychotherapy with children is not one of my own, but taken instead from *The Sixth Sense*, a 1999 supernatural thriller directed by M. Night Shyamalan. *The Sixth Sense* is one of only a handful of movies to meaningfully portray the process of child psychotherapy, though admittedly within a rather unconventional treatment framework. More pointedly, this film explores such themes as relational authenticity, self-disclosure, countertransference—and most significantly—the therapist's spontaneous tears as he reaches a treatment impasse with his young patient. In this chapter, I begin by discussing the dynamic child treatment process, and then present the case in detail. Finally, I offer tentative recommendations for how such reactions might be understood and used in the service of deepening the treatment process.

DYNAMIC CHILD PSYCHOTHERAPY

Dynamic child psychotherapy, which traces its origins to the work of such seminal psychoanalytic writers as Melanie Klein and Anna Freud, achieved wide acceptance as far back as the 1920s, originally in connection with the burgeoning child guidance movement in this country. Treatment goals in dynamic child psychotherapy include symptom resolution, the modification of behavior, some modicum of personality change, and the return of the child to a normal developmental trajectory (Sours, 1978). Child psychotherapy tends to place considerable emphasis on the child's ongoing environmental interactions independent of the treatment relationship, so that parents and siblings, school personnel, and other important figures in the child's life assume a greater importance, and may at times become directly involved in a child's treatment. While there is of course interest in the child's past, ongoing issues and conflicts are typically accorded somewhat greater significance. Regressions may occur, although the therapist, generally speaking, does not promote these.

Basic Principles of Treatment

A number of significant differences separate the psychotherapy of children from work with adults, or for that matter, with adolescents. As a general rule, few children start therapy with an expression of interest in discussing their wishes, intrapsychic conflicts, or defensive accommodations, nor are they likely to be very receptive to the therapist's efforts to introduce such ideas. This observation rests on several assumptions. The overwhelming majority of children and most adolescents do not usually seek out psychotherapy for themselves independently; rather, they are brought, sometimes quite unwillingly, into treatment by their parents. Furthermore, younger children may be uncomfortable entering into such discussions, since they have yet to acquire full mastery of spoken language and, therefore, rely far more extensively on primary process communications than do adults, who operate principally in the secondary process domain. A third factor is that the capacity for both reflective thought and for *mentalization*[2] (Fonagy & Target, 1998), may not be especially well developed in many children entering treatment.

Another difference between child and adult therapy is that children (and adolescents) are in the process of negotiating in *real time* those conflicts and crises that for the adult client are only variously accessible memories. In effect, children and adolescents are still heavily engaged with both parents and siblings in multiple discourses that for the majority of adults may have come to exist solely at the level of the imaginary. Yet another fundamental distinction lies in the repertoire of treatment techniques suitable for clinical work with either population. As I have noted, children, unlike their adolescent and adult counterparts, have yet to achieve mastery either of expressive speech or secondary process thinking and logic, so that use of the full adult range of verbalized communication is rarely possible for them (Lieberman, 1983). Thus, doll play, puppetry, modeling, therapeutic games, mud and clay, painting and drawing, computer and video games, and other "play" techniques are used either alone or (more commonly) in conjunction with elicited narratives, which, in turn, involve either direct verbal exchange or communications per metaphor.

Dynamic Listening

The narrative discourse that commences with the earliest diagnostic contact and continues throughout the entire course of a child's treatment creates a fertile environment for the evolution of the child's unique and personal story. Although in clinical assessment, a greater emphasis is placed on the historical-developmental context of a child's problems, a subtle shift must occur as the treatment process gets underway. In the first place, child treatment occurs in an *ahistorical* context, which relegates the emphasis on time and sequence and on the developmental framework that guides history taking, to assume a secondary role. Time gradually gives way to time*less*ness, which means that the rational, chronological ordering of events no longer retains its supraordinate status. Indeed, child treatment involves a continuous interweaving of themes and fantasies, and of conflict and defense, without particular attention to the logic of sequence. As I have noted, children, particularly young ones, are uncomfortable operating within the adult secondary process domain; nor are they capable of inductive or deductive logic and reasoning, instead preferring what Piaget (1969) has termed "transductive logic" (operating from particular to particular).

A more demanding task for the child therapist is creating and maintaining the necessary therapeutic ambience to enhance and promote the unfolding of the child's narrative. Permitting a child to express primitive fantasies, regressive desires, fears, or conflicts is a necessary prerequisite for such narration, although it is not sufficient. The therapist must then extract the child's story from such fragmentary and often confusing communications. It is useful to point out that even when the child's narrative seems to bear little resemblance to the historical facts, its importance is not thereby diminished. The therapist's *willing suspension of disbelief* (Coleridge, 1817/1985) in such an instance may mean the difference between mutual attunement and alliance, and therapeutic misalliance.

Understanding and responding therapeutically to the language of children's play is not altogether dissimilar to dynamic work with adult clients. Children's play and verbalized fantasies, it may be argued, bear certain fundamental similarities to the dreams of adult clients. Both are anchored in a more primitive language, that of the primary process, and therefore not typically governed by the logic and consistency of the secondary process domain. Both may be understood as possessing a *manifest* content as well as *latent* meanings, both strive for the avoidance of unpleasure or the fulfillment of wishes, and each relies heavily on the use of metaphorical and symbolic elements (although such elements, unless interpreted, generally remain outside of the subject's awareness). Finally, children's fantasies and adults' dreams may evince preoccupation with an intercurrent problem or issue, though on closer examination, sometimes also reveal earlier, historically important dynamic patterns, themes, or issues.

The clinical task of doing effective dynamic child treatment is enhanced when the therapist is alert to several key aspects of the clinical encounter. These include: the dynamic theme or issue; the representation of self and object(s) in children's play scenarios and fantasies; the child's affective tone; paralinguistic, visual, and kinesic cues; and, finally, the child's use of defensive behaviors, discrete defenses, defensive strategies, and conflict-free solutions.

- *The dynamic theme or issue.* What is the most salient issue, theme, or focal conflict in the child's communications? Childhood is filled with a range of normative problems and conflicts even when it is not disrupted by environmental crises or pathology. Various needs predominate at different phases of psychosocial and psychosexual development, encompassing everything from preschoolers' requirements for affirmation of their normal exhibitionism to the struggles of adolescents to combat the regressive pull of the nuclear family in an effort to extend their radius of social relationships. Typical focal conflicts (Brandell, 1987; Kepecs, 1977) revealed in children's fantasies, stories, and productions might include *hostility versus guilt,* the wish for *intimacy versus fear of engulfment,* the wish to be *assertive versus fear of criticism,* or the desire for *autonomy versus fear of abandonment/rejection.*

- *Representation of self and object in children's play scenarios.* Children's play and fantasies sometimes portray a unique object relational experience derived from important, affectively charged early encounters with parents, siblings, and others. Such an experience may then serve as a lens through which all subsequent object relations may be understood. For example, the fantasy narrations of a ten-year-old boy whose mother tended to be overprotective, as well as somewhat intolerant of his efforts to achieve psychological autonomy, often involved a small, rather helpless character (usually a squirrel or other small animal), dominated by a larger and more powerful character. Every autonomous effort of the smaller character was somehow thwarted or undermined by the larger one, who, like the client's mother, tended to discourage the smaller character from venturing out, being more assertive, and so forth. Even when such an object relational configuration cannot reliably be identified, it is always useful to determine which characters in play scenarios may represent the child and which character(s) appear to represent other important figures in the child's life (e.g., parents, siblings, or the therapist).

- *Affective tone.* Another important element in therapeutic play is the child's affective or hedonic tone. Does the child enter into play with interest, pleasure, vigor, and enthusiasm? Or is s/he phlegmatic, cautious, depressed, or simply going through the motions? Does the child sound mildly annoyed, angry, hurt, frustrated, anxious, agitated, fatigued, or confused? Does the child's play seem to match her/his mood, or is there a notable discrepancy?

- *Paralinguistic, visual, and kinesic cues.* Children's play is usually accompanied by a variety of sublingual utterances, distinctive facial expressions, and other, sometimes quite revealing bodily movements. Although such cues are generally consonant with the play themes and actions, they are at other times rather asynchronous or poorly matched. For instance, a very depressed nine-year-old girl, whose father abandoned the family, had quite a fanciful imagination. Her fantasy play often involved larger-than-life characters that embarked on high adventures in exotic locales. At the same time, her manner was remarkable for its *economy* of movement, and she looked and sounded depressed, her demeanor at striking variance with the content and themes of her play.

- *The child's defensive behaviors, discrete defenses, defensive strategies, and conflict-free solutions.* Children's play narrations often contain compromise solutions to conflict, typically activated by the ego's defensive function, which recognizes the danger of direct expression or fulfillment of a disturbing wish and seeks to disguise it in some manner. These accommodations include defensive behaviors in very young children (e.g., transformation of affect), discrete defenses (e.g., denial, undoing, isolation, or withdrawal), and wishes used defensively (e.g., hostility directed against the self, defensive intimacy, or defensive assertion). Relatively conflict-free adaptive strategies emerge as the child acquires more capacity for self-observation and insight, usually during the latter phases of treatment.

TEARS IN CHILD PSYCHOTHERAPY

A Child's Tears

Child clients may be moved to tears for a variety of reasons in the psychotherapy encounter. Thematically, certain issues, such as parental divorce and separation, life-threatening illness of a close family member, and of course the loss of a parent, sibling, or other close relative or friend, may be likely to educe tearful reactions in children, both within and outside of therapy. Children who are experiencing psychological, physical, or sexual abuse, or neglect, may, at times, become tearful in therapy, as may those who have been subject to bullying at school or elsewhere. Children who present with various kinds of depressive problems, as well as those with symptoms of anxiety, or who have developed psychological problems secondary to physical health conditions, might also be moved to tears in a psychotherapy session. More seriously disturbed children, such as those who suffer from self-object disorders (Tolpin & Kohut, 1980) and nascent forms of characterological disturbance, and thus have difficulty regulating their affective reactions, might also be more likely to react with tears during the course of a therapy session. As discussed earlier, the clinical milieu in child treatment can be quite different from that in work with adult clients, in good measure owing to the relative preponderance of primary process communications. However, in an important sense, the strength of certain affective reactions a child registers in the course of a therapy session may have an existence that is largely independent of his or her diagnosis or predisposing circumstances. Put somewhat differently, children don't need to be "disturbed" to cry in therapy; at various times, as certain play themes or issues evoke strong affective reactions, being moved to tears may be the most natural, if not, universal reaction. Such emotions might include (but are hardly limited to) grief, sadness, anger, rage, anxiety, fear, shame, bewilderment, excitement, exuberance, and pleasure.

A Therapist's Tears

Almost equally, there are a number of situations in which a child therapist might possibly be moved to tears in working with a client. Certain types of clients might be more likely to evoke such reactions from their therapists, generally speaking: children suffering from life-threatening health conditions, those experiencing deep depression or despair, child victims of profound neglect or abuse, and children who have suffered severe traumas are certainly among this group. A therapist's tears might also signify a more *classical* countertransference reaction, as in the case of a child whose conflicts or behavior have re-stimulated the therapist's own unworked-through issues. Additional possibilities are that the therapist has reacted with frustration to a child's resistant behavior, or is crying *for* a child who is incapable of summoning this affect him or herself. Yet another possibility is that the therapist tears up spontaneously as an expression of relief, or of pride in the client's accomplishments. We must remember that tears may also signify pleasure, as when one is deeply moved by a beautiful piece of orchestral music, or a work of art, or a poetic passage in a literary work. More pointedly, we may cry upon hearing the long-awaited revelation of a repressed and resistant client, or at the moment a withdrawn client begins to emerge from her protective cocoon, or a dependent, helpless client takes the first steps toward autonomy and mastery. And, of course, we also cry *with* our child clients, just as we do with our adult clients, at times of great sadness or triumph, or other outpourings of raw emotion, in what could be described as a spontaneous, concordant countertransference reaction (Racker, 1968).

In the classical child psychoanalytic literature, to the extent it was even discussed, countertransference represented a hindrance to the productive work of therapy. Indeed, as Kohrman, Fineberg, Gelman, and Weiss reported in a 1971 article, a treatment focus on the manifestations and meanings of countertransference was at that time largely regarded as being "off-limits."[3] With the ascendancy of a two-person psychoanalytic psychology and the influence of relational theory, this position has gradually been modified in recent years. Arguably, the therapist's tears, much like her/his other subjective reactions, potentially may possess both diagnostic and therapeutic value. One might even conceive of such emotional reactions as constituting a "facilitative" condition (Rogers, 1957) for effective child treatment, insofar as the therapist's tearful reactions may signify empathy, congruence, and/or genuineness. It is, of course, also possible that the therapist's tears may have an inhibitory effect, or even prove frightening to a child. For example, a child who has served as a source of emotional support for a severely depressed parent, or who is otherwise "parentified," may feel that s/he needs to enact a similar posture with the therapist. Obviously, in such an instance, with its implied reversal of roles, treatment may easily become derailed. Therefore, trying to establish "ground rules" for how one manages such tearful reactions may be difficult, if not impossible, owing to the infinite variation that exists among child clients and the specific circumstances of their treatment.

That having been said, it is easy to imagine specific scenarios where the therapist's tears may have a catalytic effect on a treatment that has reached an impasse, or with a child who has been raised in an emotionally repressive home environment. Such a reaction in the therapist may anticipate a child's own suppressed sorrow, and thereby make possible the expression of grief that has been partially or wholly outside the child's own awareness or otherwise defended against. It may also serve as a sort of bridge to traumatic memories from which the original affective reactions have become separated. For example, traumatized children may be able to recall the events surrounding a traumatic experience, but in an incomplete and dissociated form. The therapist's spontaneous affective response to the child's revelations furnishes what has been missing from such traumatic memories, offering a pathway to healing that even the most carefully timed and accurate interpretations may fall short of providing. Whether such tearful reactions are acknowledged, discussed, or explored in greater depth is perhaps best left to the therapist's discretion, as would other kinds of emotional reactions or instances of countertransference.

Clinical Illustration: *The Sixth Sense*

As this story begins, Dr. Malcolm Crowe (Bruce Willis), a 40-ish child psychologist, has just returned home from a romantic evening of celebration with his adoring wife, Anna. Unbeknownst to them, a patient whom Dr. Crowe had treated as a child some 12 years earlier has broken into their home, and waits silently in an upstairs bathroom clad only in his undershorts. Vincent

Grey, the former patient, is barely coherent and enraged when he confronts Dr. Crowe. He bitterly accuses his former therapist of the profoundest insensitivity and emotional betrayal, but before Dr. Crowe is able to respond, Vincent shoots him and then suicides by turning the gun on himself. Eight or nine months pass, during which Dr. Crowe, healing from the gunshot, becomes obsessed with this case and its tragic outcome. Despite the fact that his mantelpiece is adorned with thank-you notes from grateful young patients and his high professional competence and dedication are formally acknowledged in a special award given to him by the city of Philadelphia, he feels little pride. This dramatic treatment failure and the endless ruminations to which it gives rise have nullified all his prior accomplishments. In the aftermath of the trauma, his work and his marriage are both affected. Dr. Crowe pores over his notes from Vincent's treatment, searching for answers that continue to elude him.

Still not fully recovered, he takes on a new patient. Cole Sear (Haley Joel Osment), like Vincent at the time he began therapy, is in mid-latency and unusually compassionate; in other respects, too, he is uncannily reminiscent of Dr. Crowe's earlier patient. In the remainder of the film, Dr. Crowe and his young patient confront their respective demons, and a poignant therapeutic encounter between a traumatized boy and his traumatized therapist is gradually revealed.

Cole is a bright, sensitive boy who lives in a small apartment with his mother. His father evidently has abandoned the family several years earlier, and Cole and his mother struggle to survive on whatever income she is able to generate from working long hours at two jobs. Cole has two cherished possessions that once belonged to his father: a pair of eyeglasses (which he wears in the beginning of the film *sans* lenses because the lenses hurt his eyes), and a wristwatch that no longer works that he discovered in his father's drawer. Cole's relationship with his dad, like the empty frames and the stopped wristwatch, seems as ghostly as the apparitions he claims to see. Chronological time has ceased to have meaning in Cole's life, for his own pain and disappointments have become gradually commingled with the tragedies that extrude, hauntingly, into his consciousness. Cole is metaphorically suspended in the twilight intersection of past and present, neither capable of reflecting on the meaning of what has been nor able to imagine what may come.

In the first encounter between Dr. Crowe and his youthful patient, which takes place in a Catholic church, Cole's posttraumatic play provides Dr. Crowe with a glimpse of the madness that this small boy carries within. What the viewer witnesses is a joyless, driven play scenario, more on the order of a compulsive re-enactment rather than the healthy creativity of the primary process, the language of fantasy play, that one might ordinarily expect to see in a child of Cole's age. One of the small icons Cole plays with in a dimly lit pew is a tortured soldier who utters the Latin phrase *"De profundus clamo ad Te Domine"* ("Out of the depths, I cry to you, Oh Lord"). Dr. Crowe is immediately fascinated by this case, deeply motivated by his wish to understand and help this child find a pathway leading out of his profound despair and pain. But Cole has a secret that he is not at first prepared to share, not even with this dedicated and compassionate therapist. Cole has little reason to believe that Dr. Crowe has anything to offer that is substantively different from the other adults in his life. Like so many children, Cole has concluded that the truth is dangerous and off-putting for adults and, perhaps more significantly, that most adults are far less interested in listening to children than they may at first claim. Rather, their interests are in having children conform to the rules, in directing their play and work, offering advice and guidance, or perhaps simply in hearing themselves speak. Cole no longer draws pictures of the ghastly images he sees, since it proved far too disturbing for the staff at his school. "I draw pictures of rainbows and dogs running," he says. "They don't have meetings about rainbows." It is, of course, no surprise that Cole begins to feel freakish, for his distrust includes peers, as well: no one, it seems, can be entrusted with his awesome secret.

It is only after Dr. Crowe has convincingly demonstrated his commitment to Cole that Cole can begin to describe the ineffable. From his hospital bed, at a critical juncture in the beginning of a real therapeutic alliance between patient and therapist, Cole whispers to Dr. Crowe, "I see dead people." It is significant that Dr. Crowe, though moved by Cole's painful struggle, is not at first able to believe Cole's story. With great resignation, he views Cole as more disturbed than he had originally thought, a paranoid child subject to powerful visual hallucinations who appears to be suffering from some sort of "school-age schizophrenia." He begins to consider the possibility that drugs or hospitalization may be required, all the while sounding more and more distant. As he focuses increasingly on Cole's symptomatology, the objectification of his young patient seems to be leading Dr. Crowe to the inevitability of repeating his earlier error with Vincent.

Soon Dr. Crowe realizes the dilemma with which he is confronted. Though he wants desperately to help Cole, he feels powerless in the face of this boy's terrifying psychotic-like symptoms. He cannot accept Cole's description of his paranormal experiences, and yet without being able to take this step, to believe what Cole tells him, Dr. Crowe is unable to join his patient as an ally in this nightmare world. Helpless and frightened, Dr. Crowe tells Cole that he is not able to meet with him any longer, and that he will be transferring his case. Cole, facing yet another abandonment, feels more alone than ever. He beseeches Dr. Crowe to reconsider this decision, arguing that Dr. Crowe is the only one who can help him. It is at this moment that Dr. Crowe's eyes begin to fill with tears. Cole begins to cry now, as well, but accurately surmises that his therapist is deeply conflicted over the decision he has just announced to transfer Cole's case. Perhaps sensing that Dr. Crowe's tears signify the true emotional investment he feels for Cole's therapy, Cole asks something that we imagine he has never asked anyone before: "You believe me, right?" When Dr. Crowe is unable to respond, Cole poses a critically important question: "How can you help me if you don't believe me?"

In this scene, the unremitting pain both therapist and child feel becomes almost palpable. Dr. Crowe's tragic treatment failure with Vincent looms so large that it has gradually overshadowed his successes with so many others, leaving him wounded and filled with self-doubt, no longer able to believe in himself or his skills as a therapist nor even capable of finding solace in his marriage. Cole's abandonment by his father and social ostracism by peers have created a painful inner emptiness that amplifies the sense of freakishness he feels due to his paranormal abilities. He is overcome by an abiding sense of powerlessness and hopelessness. He is haunted, however, not only by his own past but also by the unfathomable pain and bitterness of the spectral beings that seek him out, souls whose human lives have ended unfairly, starkly, and in tragedy.

In an important sense, both Cole and Dr. Crowe are caught in the timelessness of their pasts; each requires the other in order to establish a new *telos*, and to plot the trajectory that will lead to a final resolution. "Therapist" and "patient," therefore, become rather ambiguous roles as this treatment alliance begins to cohere. Dr. Crowe learns about a spectral order from a boy who sees and hears things that he cannot; ironically, he is able to show his young friend a new way of listening and communing with the very souls whose existence the therapist was initially unable to accept. In this fundamentally intersubjective and evolutionary process, Dr. Crowe, the wounded healer, also acquires the strength and insight to confront painful truths that he himself has disavowed for many months, if not longer. (And, in fact, it is through this personal journey of the therapist that the movie offers up its final, shocking plot twist.)

Interestingly, Dr. Crowe's personal struggle to help Cole is always obvious to both patient and doctor. At one point, Dr. Crowe, speaking to Cole per metaphor, describes his earlier work with Vincent, making an allusion to its poor outcome; the possibility that he may be helpful to Cole, Dr. Crowe continues, represents a second chance, an opportunity to wrest meaning from tragedy and professional defeat. Several times, Dr. Crowe tries somewhat half-heartedly to evade Cole's questions to him about his personal life, but Cole's feelings and insights about his therapist are unerringly accurate; Dr. Crowe is compelled to speak of his troubled marriage, perhaps even with a sense of relief. Does such spontaneous self-disclosure bode poorly for the treatment process? Apparently it does not. Although Dr. Crowe has a powerful personal agenda from his very first encounter with Cole, his professional concern and an abiding love for his patient appear finally to guide his clinical decisions. Not all of these decisions are correct, however, and one, in particular, represents a glaring error.

That error is Dr. Crowe's resistance to accepting the importance of his patient's narrative, which follows Cole's hospital-bed revelation, "I see dead people." As previously suggested, when Dr. Crowe begins to think of Cole as a very disturbed child, or perhaps more accurately, as a collection of disturbing, psychotic-like symptoms, he removes himself from the intersubjective field, which both therapist and child experience as alienating. What is especially interesting about the scene in which Dr. Crowe tells Cole he must transfer his case is the fact that something inside of him, a powerful emotional reaction to this child, seems to belie the conventional clinical wisdom he uses to justify the proposed transfer to another therapist. It is as if Dr. Crowe's tears signify a relationally authentic part of himself that he attempts to suppress.

Interestingly, just as Dr. Crowe is beginning to question his small patient's sense of reality, Cole's apparitions become visible for us, the audience. Perhaps this is intended to signify the new meaning these ghostly images acquire through Cole's profound admission to his therapist. They have become more real, acquiring visual form because Cole has described them and made them a part of his treatment. It now becomes Dr. Crowe's task to accept as a verisimilitude what Cole has revealed to him without dismissing such paranormal experiences as the hallucinations of a psychotic child. This is not, of course, easily accomplished either in real life or in good movies. In this instance, Dr. Crowe can only permit himself to be convinced of what Cole tells him after returning to an audiotape of an interview with Vincent made a dozen years earlier. Because Cole has taught him how to listen and what to listen for, he hears things that have always been there but that had previously eluded him. Suddenly, Cole's fantastic claims are no longer as frightening, and a significant therapeutic breach has been repaired. Enlightened, Dr. Crowe is able to re-enter Cole's world, and a real therapeutic process begins.

Let us return for a moment to the critical scene during which Dr. Crowe tells Cole he must transfer his case to another therapist. It is my belief that Dr. Crowe's tears reveal an important aspect of his countertransference to this deeply troubled child patient. I am here defining countertransference rather broadly, to represent the totality of a therapist's subjective reactions, both conscious and unconscious, educed from the therapist in the context of ongoing therapeutic work with a client. Further, such reactions may consist of fantasies, thoughts, attitudes, affects, counterreactions, counterresistances, behavior, and behavioral enactments (Brandell, 2004). Dr. Crowe's tears are but one aspect of his more encompassing subjective experience of the client, but in addition, they touch on an aspect of his earlier treatment failure with Vincent, the former patient who committed suicide after shooting Dr. Crowe. Countertransference, of course, may also involve displacements of affective or ideational phenomena from historically important relationships of the therapist. This would seem very much to be the case for Dr. Crowe, whose preoccupation with Vincent's failed treatment cannot but influence his inability to make therapeutic progress with Cole Sear.

Dr. Crowe's tears may simultaneously represent the above-referenced displacement, his own sense of inadequacy with Cole, and the expression of a deep affective resonance with Cole's pain and psychological distress. Dr. Crowe only tears up for a moment, quickly regaining his composure as this session with his emotionally distraught client comes to an end. It has been noted in the child treatment literature that the concept of countertransference was largely neglected prior to the 1980s, even as there was a burgeoning interest in the topic as it pertains to adult treatment (Brandell, 1992). Various explanations have been offered for this curious disparity, ranging from the failure of child therapy pioneers such as Melanie Klein and Anna Freud to address the phenomenon, to the dyssynchrony of countertransference with the universal value in protecting, nurturing, and giving guidance to young children (Brandell, 1992).

Phenomenologically speaking, self-disclosure is closely related to the topic of countertransference. Self-disclosure may be reflexive and largely unconscious, as, for example, in slips of the tongue, errors of commission or omission, or other non-verbal phenomena outside the therapist's conscious awareness (Brandell, 2004). On the other hand, self-disclosures may represent deliberate actions, as, for example, the decision to share various subjective experiences, or to respond to a client's questions or requests for personal information from the therapist (Strean, 2002). The therapist's expression of tearful affect seems to be a particularly clear example of a spontaneously arising self-disclosure.

Actually, it appears that Dr. Crowe's tears disclose something that his words do not; his tears, indeed, appear to be at variance with his words, and convey a fundamental dyssynchrony to Cole. While his stated objective is to transfer Cole's case to a colleague, Dr. Crowe's tears reveal the depth of his continuing emotional investment in the boy's case, evidence of just how profoundly Cole has affected him. As noted previously, Cole appears to be moved by his doctor's emotional response, perhaps seeing his tears as proof of the therapist's deep continuing concern for him. Such an announcement (i.e., the intention to transfer or terminate a case), even when delivered in an attuned and clinically even-handed manner, is nevertheless, fundamentally experienced as an abandonment. In less-than-ideal circumstances, therapeutic transfers and forced terminations are experienced as microtraumas, and have the potential to engender such strong reactions as acting out, rage, significant regressions, and withdrawal, depression, or even despair. Cole, however, is unwilling to accept the verbal message he has just received, and instead, continues to engage Dr. Crowe by asking him for his help and by seeking his trust. Cole's ability to remain emotionally engaged, facilitated, I believe, by his doctor's tears, ultimately enlivens what had threatened to become a moribund treatment. While Dr. Crowe's and Cole's tears signify something unique to each, their tears also represent an intersubjective phenomenon, attesting on some level to the pain that they share and the connection they feel to one another.

CONCLUSION AND RECOMMENDATIONS

This chapter has explored the topic of the therapist's tearful reactions to child clients, beginning with a general review of some basic principles of dynamic child psychotherapy, followed by a discussion of the clinical significance of both children's and therapist's tears, and the meanings such emotional reactions possess and convey in the child therapy treatment milieu. The chapter concludes with a detailed clinical illustration derived from the popular media.

The clinical illustration I used was taken from Shyamalan's 1999 supernatural thriller, *The Sixth Sense*, a story about an extraordinary encounter between a therapist and a child. In part because this story is so well told, but also because it permits us *entrée* to the intersubjective field of child therapist and client, it offers us valuable lessons about the nature of healing that clinical journals, textbooks, and modern-day practice too often neglect. Dr. Crowe's tearful reaction, aside from signaling a deep emotional synchrony with this youthful client, also reveals his growing frustration in being unable to help Cole. Additionally, it represents the recrudescence of his earlier therapeutic failure with Vincent. Dr. Crowe doesn't discuss his reaction with Cole, but it appears to serve as a key factor in his enhanced understanding of this very troubled client. This new understanding then permits him to work through his own trauma, thereby enriching Cole's treatment in the process. Dr. Crowe, the wounded healer, has regained a capacity for listening, though with far greater depth than he had previously been capable. Of equal importance is that when Dr. Crowe's eyes well up with tears, it not only makes possible Cole's *own* tearful reaction, but it also offers Cole proof of Dr. Crowe's deep affective commitment to Cole's case, thus enabling him to pose vital questions to his doctor. In this sense, the treatment is truly intersubjective, a therapeutic encounter in which two subjects, each with a unique history, and conflicted wishes and desires, acts on the other.

For reasons discussed above, it is rather challenging to present specific guidelines or recommendations to child therapists on the subject of the therapist's tearful reactions to a child client. Nevertheless, a few general recommendations are possible:

1. Although the open expression of tearful affect (and of countertransference reactions, more generally) would likely have been discouraged within a traditional psychodynamic framework, contemporary psychodynamic theory tends to view the treatment relationship as a two-person encounter that privileges genuineness and relational authenticity. Therefore, such reactions are regarded as being neither bad nor good, but rather as offering *potential*.
2. Tearful affect, like most countertransference reactions of the therapist, has informational value. Such information may pertain to the client, to the therapist's self, or to aspects of the treatment relationship, but always warrants self-reflection and understanding.
3. Child clients deserve to have the therapist acknowledge any strong affective reaction, though the explanation can be simple, and needn't include details the client would find burdensome.
4. It is also possible for a therapist to acknowledge a tearful reaction, but defer discussion to a later time.

NOTES

1. Portions of this chapter are drawn from two earlier publications of the author: "Listening at the Movies," an essay which appeared in *Readings,* March 2000, *15*(1), 6–11, a publication of the American Orthopsychiatric Association; and *Of Mice and Metaphors: Therapeutic Storytelling with Children,* published in 2000 by Basic Books.

2. *Mentalization* has been defined as the ability to create and make use of mental representations of one's own and others' emotional states (Fonagy & Target, 1998).
3. Kohrman et al. refer anecdotally to an experience that one of the authors had while participating in a clinical discussion of a child analytic case at a national conference. This therapist had suggested at an opportune moment that a puzzling aspect of the case under discussion might be illuminated by examining the therapist's contributions to the clinical situation, which appeared to signal a possible countertransference issue. At this point, the moderator intervened, declaring emphatically, "We don't talk about such things" (1971, p. 488).

REFERENCES

Brandell, J. (1987). Focal conflict theory: A model for teaching dynamic practice. *Social Casework, 68*, 299–310.

Brandell, J. (Ed.) (1992). *Countertransference in psychotherapy with children and adolescents*. Northvale, NJ: Jason Aronson.

Brandell, J. (2000, March). Listening at the movies. *Readings, 15*(1), 6–11.

Brandell, J. (2000). *Of mice and metaphors: Therapeutic storytelling with children*. New York, NY: Basic Books.

Brandell, J. (2004). *Psychodynamic social work*. New York, NY: Columbia University Press.

Coleridge, S. (1817/1985). Biographia literaria. In H. J. Jackson (Ed.). *Samuel Taylor Coleridge: The major works* (pp. 155–482). Oxford, UK: Oxford University Press.

Fonagy, P., & Target, M. (1998). Mentalization and the changing aims of child psychoanalysis. *Psychoanalytic Dialogues, 8*, 87–114.

Kepecs, J. (1977). Teaching psychotherapy by use of brief transcripts. *American Journal of Psychotherapy, 31*, 383–393.

Kohrman, R., Fineberg, H., Gelman, R., & Weiss, S. (1971). Technique of child analysis: Problems of countertransference. *The International Journal of Psycho-Analysis, 59*, 487–497.

Lieberman, F. (1983). Work with children. In D. Waldfogel & A. Rosenblatt (Eds.), *Handbook of clinical social work* (pp. 441–465). San Francisco, CA: Jossey-Bass.

Piaget, J. (1969). *The psychology of the child*. New York, NY: Basic Books.

Racker, H. (1968). *Transference and countertransference*. New York, NY: International Universities Press.

Rogers, C. (1957). The necessary and sufficient conditions of therapeutic personality change. *Journal of Consulting Psychology, 22,* 95–103.

Shyamalan, M. (Director), & Marshall, F., Kennedy, K., Mendel, B. (Producers). (1999). *The sixth sense* [motion picture]. United States: Buena Vista/Hollywood/Spyglass.

Sours, J. (1978). The application of child analytic principles to forms of child psychotherapy. In J. Glenn (Ed.), *Child analysis and therapy* (pp. 615–646). New York, NY: Jason Aronson.

Strean, H. (2002). Countertransference: An introduction. In H. Strean (Ed.), *Controversies on countertransference* (pp. 1–24). Northvale, NJ: Jason Aronson.

Tolpin, M., & Kohut, H. (1980). The disorders of the self: The psychopathology of the first years of life. In S. Greenspan & G. Pollock (Eds.), *The course of life: Psychoanalytic contributions toward understanding personality development* (pp. 425–442). Rockville, MD: National Institute of Mental Health.

CHAPTER 13

TEARS OF THE EMERGING PARENT: THERAPISTS' TEARS IN WORKING WITH PREGNANT AND POSTPARTUM CLIENTS

Wendy N. Davis

> *"You're crying," she says quietly, leaning forward in her chair ever so slightly. She looks at me across the space, and her face relaxes for the first time since we began our session. We let the moment be: the quiet, my tears, the last sun coming in the window, and then the cloud that takes its place. Our eye contact feels easy and does not falter. I don't wipe my tears, and she doesn't cry, but her eyes soften. She pauses in the telling of her story, and we sit in the moment, leaving space for the potential of connection, acknowledgment, and relief. Eventually, I nod. "Yes," I say, "I'm listening to what you've been going through."*

Jill[1] began counseling with me soon after her daughter was born, referred by her doctor after Jill talked of feeling increasingly depressed and anxious. When she paused in response to my tears, allowing herself to feel the depth of her own story, I felt gratitude: a familiar but spontaneous appreciation for the courage and grace present when a client takes the risk of sharing and feeling her pain, and ventures the tender steps toward hope and healing. In that moment after my own tears, Jill decided to share her story fully, despite the judgment and alienation she had felt in her attempts to share with others before. With trust that perhaps came from the compassion my tears showed her, she risked my judgment or misunderstanding or potential further alienation. In that moment, she trusted me to listen and trusted herself to withstand the pain, grief, and suffering. She trusted that there would be solid ground for her to move forward upon. I ask myself often: how can I best help in these brave first steps forward? In Jill's case, do my tears in our early session make her self-conscious, more afraid of the deep reservoir of sadness within her? Or do they aid her, attesting to the fact that pain has occurred, but that healing will also take place? I don't ask Jill in that moment. It would feel intrusive to insert the question into the space between us. It is her moment, and my tears should be quiet and natural in the room, not something to announce, but more light rain on the window.

Later, I do ask her: "How did my tears affect you?" She recounts that very process of stepping into the unknown, describing a new world that she imagines might hold love and freedom, but in the moment presents a terrifying step. For Jill, her old world was shadowed by criticism and shame from her family of origin, a world of derision that she had occupied for her whole life without full awareness of how painful it was. Becoming a parent brought this old dynamic into stark relief. The process of therapy helped her to see that world for what it was, and to come into a new world that gave her a much fuller, more loving view of herself, her life, and her new family. In a letter Jill sent to me regarding the meaning of tears in the six-year process of our psychotherapy, which she gave me permission to share, she describes how my tears in in our first session gave her a sense of hope:

> *A lot of therapy for me has been this process of stepping over from one world to another. Step by step, it has taken such a long time, from a whole different universe where all the rules were different, and nothing ever made sense but I always had to try try try—and even though that world was made up of eight people in my childhood family, and I'm stepping over into the actual world, into reality, with everyone else, with all that means, still it felt like blind groping into something that might not exist for a very long time. Your tears showed that it did, that there was a different world waiting.*

In this chapter, I describe important aspects of therapeutic work with pregnant and postpartum clients. I then discuss therapists' tears in therapy when doing this work, concluding by offering recommendations for practice.

WORKING WITH PREGNANT AND POSTPARTUM CLIENTS

In the life of pregnant and postpartum women and their partners, there are many kinds of tears. There are the tears of the baby, and there are the tears of the parent. The woman who comes to counseling has experienced floods of tears: tears of frustration, sadness, despair, exhaustion, and grief. If you ask, you might hear about her partner's tears, a silent accompaniment to the stress in the family. And further back, as therapy reveals, perhaps there are memories of her mother's tears, or her own tears as a child.

Many mothers relay chaotic times at home when suddenly everyone is crying and all seems upside down with stress, angst, and exhaustion. When she comes to therapy, she now has a quiet place and perhaps a new experience of crying, one of release and relief, a connection with a caring guide. Here, her tears are not the cloudburst between her and her baby or partner, but they are a part of her connecting with her own experience. When the therapist also sheds tears in these moments, there is a very important difference between the therapist's tears and the tears of others in the client's life: in a healthy and centered therapeutic relationship, the therapist's tears have no sting. I am not crying out of frustration or angst. I am not hurt. I am not in despair. I am connecting, feeling compassion, having a spontaneous human reaction born of empathy and moved by the moment when suffering is revealed.

Experts define perinatal mood and anxiety disorders by symptoms of emotional distress that begin during pregnancy or any time through the first year postpartum. Women of every culture, age, income level, and race can develop perinatal mood and anxiety disorders, and are more vulnerable to mental health disorders around the time of childbearing than at any other time in their lives (Eaton et al., 2012). Although postpartum depression (PPD) has been described as the most common complication of childbearing (Brealey, Hewitt, Green, Morrell, & Gilbody, 2010), it often goes unrecognized and not fully treated, even when new parents are engaged in therapy. When a mental health provider begins to suspect PPD in a client, she or he usually looks for sadness and lack of feeling toward the baby. However, just as often, mothers with a perinatal mental health crisis are highly anxious, striving to be perfect, hiding their most difficult thoughts and feelings even from their therapists, all while holding on to their own interpretation that they are failing as a parent. While we mostly hear about PPD, we now understand that there are a variety of perinatal mood and anxiety disorders. The most effective prevention, assessment, treatment, and education recognize all of the distinct mental health conditions common to pregnancy and the postpartum period: depression, anxiety, obsessive-compulsive disorder, posttraumatic stress, bipolar disorders, and psychosis (Meltzer-Brody, 2011).

Beyond the natural period of adjustment experienced by all parents, research shows at least one in seven women will experience significant depression or anxiety during or after pregnancy (Wisner et al., 2013). Perhaps more surprisingly, large-scale studies by the American Academy of Pediatrics found that as many as 10% of new fathers also have depression or anxiety following childbirth (Paulson & Bazemore, 2010). Besides postpartum mood disorders, perinatal mental health counseling also includes struggles with fertility, pregnancy loss, stillbirth, and the fears that come with subsequent pregnancy after a loss. Further, for many women, the profound shifts of pregnancy, childbirth, and postpartum life unexpectedly bring memories of trauma, abuse, and new grief from previous losses. New or expectant mothers and fathers often come to therapy after newly erupted traumatic memories. This is a profound opportunity for discovery, healing, and recovery, and the compassionate witnessing of the therapeutic guide is essential in that process.

Every baby enters an environment with a unique interplay of their needs and caregiver response, comfort and discomfort, attachment and development. We know that the mental health and emotional well-being of parents are crucial parts of that environment, but we are still learning how to talk about that in ways that encourage strength and recovery rather than triggering shame and fear. Despite advances in understanding pregnancy and postpartum mental health and increased public awareness of PPD, it is still very difficult for new parents to recognize signs and symptoms in themselves when they occur. Most often, the struggling new or expecting parent sees him- or herself as failing, feels frightened, and is embarrassed to reach out for the help that is so vital to recovery. Counseling with the perinatal population is one way to create a safe place for parents to experience and move through their grief, anxiety, and isolation. The compassionate response of the therapist, including tears when moved, is part of that new and honest space. My tears often surprise me in this very moment; that is, when I reflect to my clients the strength, grace, and resilience that they are using as a new mother or father, but that they themselves do not yet see.

Acknowledgment of despair is absent in our cultural conversations about childbearing and parenthood. Instead, media and marketing show new parents sweet and delicate images of mommies and babies, and there is a relative taboo against sharing the experience of sadness and grief during "the happiest time of your life." New and expecting parents are thrust unexpectedly into a world of isolation and shame when they find themselves depressed, anxious, and experiencing scary thoughts or mood swings. It is from the sense of failure and isolation that a client might enter therapy.

Working with pregnancy and postpartum mental health, there are so many natural situations to inspire tears. Perinatal mood disorders are only one of the many reasons that crying occurs for new mothers. In fact, the time of pregnancy, childbirth, postpartum, and perinatal loss is one of the most vulnerable life transitions, both in the prevalence of mental health disorders, but also in the profound emotional, social, and spiritual experiences of pregnancy, childbirth, and new parenthood. Indeed, in a study of what makes adults cry, the birth of a child is first on the list (Vingerhoets & Bylsma, 2015).

TEARS IN THERAPY WITH THE EMERGING PARENT

Working With Jill: The Evolving Meaning of Tears

When Jill came to her first session, I expected to begin a therapeutic relationship familiar to me as a specialist: the journey of discovery, understanding, and recovery with the postpartum mom or dad whose expectations of parenthood have been shattered by the shock and stress of a mental health crisis at this vulnerable time. In fact, as it so often happens, my expectation was met with the power and individuality of her story as it unfolded. As a therapist, it is a common experience to have your expectations fall by the wayside if you are really listening to the person in front of you. Skilled therapists know that it is their job to be present for the unfolding, to not know what to expect, even to allow themselves to feel blank and "not-smart," so that they can really listen. It is from this openness that a true response emerges, and that response might be when tears appear. I experience my therapy tears as if I am listening to the most poignant piece of music, and I cry in the same way. Quietly, so I don't miss the music.

I learned that Jill's doctor had given her my name a year before our first session. Although it is not unusual for people to take a long time to call, in her case the reason was profound. A year earlier, Jill and her husband lost their first child at birth. She gave birth to a precious and stillborn baby boy who would always be their first child. They had been referred to a specialist in perinatal loss just after the birth, but came away feeling worse, alienated by the sense that their authentic experience was not heard or seen. In the face of their raw and craggy grief, the counseling felt prescribed and scripted. They agreed that they felt better talking to one another, and Jill was very hesitant to seek counseling again. But now it was a year later, they had a new baby girl, and Jill was struggling.

When I was a new therapist, I likely would have been deeply affected and even moved to tears just hearing about her first loss. But that is not what made me cry with Jill. On reflection of my own process over time, I understand something about the development of my therapeutic tears. It is not the client's sadness, or my own, that makes me cry; it is not just the loss. Yes, I feel deep sadness hearing about her first childbirth experience, but my tears come more from empathy and compassion than from sympathy. The empathic response connects me all at once to pathos and to the client. When I pay attention to what is actually happening within me, it is truly a sweet feeling to experience that resonance; I experience it as if a fresh breeze just came through the room, opening up the space and connecting us.

As therapists, we process information on many levels at once. No matter what I am feeling as a sympathetic response or in my assumptions about my client's experience, I have learned to focus on my pure observations and let my clients fill the room with their truth. It is my task to help that truth unfold; I am at my best when I listen, observe, and respect the unique experience of my client. When I relinquished my own expectations about Jill and the experience of stillbirth, I noticed that when she talked about her firstborn, a look of peace came over her. *She still loves that child.* It was as if a light turned on and her spirit lifted for a moment. I could hear that Jill and her husband worked hard emotionally and spiritually through that delivery and loss and in their attempt to find support, and she was indeed able to find a place of peace through the birth and death process.

In the early session with Jill described at this start of this chapter, what brought forth my tears was witnessing this striving new mother, who had gracefully navigated one of the most difficult experiences one can imagine, now feel that she was failing. She was overcome with a growing depression and anxiety under the weight of self-criticism, and a yet-to-be-understood pattern of emotional abuse from her family of origin. My tears came as I listened to her story: how she tried to reach out to her family after the loss of their firstborn and again through this new pregnancy, only to be accosted by their criticism and ridicule. With another family, this wise and loving couple might have completed a profound grief process and been supported by their family as the resilient parents they were. Instead, Jill's attempts to search for the loving embrace of her family resulted in a depressing weekly ritual of lengthy belittling phone calls and emails with her mother and sister that tore away at her potential recovery and healing as a new mother. Instead of the encouraging words one would hope the new mom would receive in her grief and recovery, her family chided her for talking about the stillbirth and "being so morbid." Then, after her new baby was safely born, Jill's mother and sister criticized her for not looking like herself: "We looked for a picture of you in that online folder you sent, but all we saw was an ugly woman and her baby. That wasn't you, was it?" Jill would finish each call with great sadness and anxiety.

In our early sessions, Jill was not yet conscious of the emotional effect of her mother's and sister's words. Even as she related stories of isolation and humiliation as a child, and described current conversations with her mother and sister in which I could hear the sharp devaluing and undermining, she could not understand why she felt like such a failure after talking to them. "I'm really close to them. I just don't know why I keep feeling worse. What's wrong with me? Maybe I shouldn't have been a mother." Perhaps her mind was not able to fully process the long-standing pattern of verbal abuse or hear it anew in these vulnerable times. She wondered why she was struggling each week, when she had "so much support."

When you become a new parent, it is not uncommon for issues from family of origin to resurface. This is a time when so many people want to turn to a parent or family member(s) for support and, in an ideal world, who better for a new mother to turn to for guidance about parenting than her own mother? However, when Jill turned to her mother, she became entrapped in the toxic, devaluing dynamic that she had been embedded in as a child, causing her to feel familiar feelings of failure, this time in her role as a parent. And what is worse than a new mother feeling that her own mother disapproves of her as a parent? On top of that, the failure mothers can irrationally feel after losing a child to stillbirth burdened Jill with another layer of self-criticism and doubt that she could not quite explain. The family dynamic she was subject to in her interactions with her mother and sister was not yet clear to her and her painful emotions around the loss of her firstborn were still so raw. My tears in our early session showed her that I was not criticizing a woman who was failing her children, but that I was feeling with, and moved by, the strength and resilience of a woman who was not a failure, despite all of this. My tears, at first, cried feelings that Jill herself could not yet feel. Later, my tears joined hers as a sign that she was not alone. As Jill came to recognize the painful dynamic with her mother and sister, she was eventually able to dispute the criticism and fight the feelings of failure that plagued her. In a sense, as she came to realize that it was her own mother who had failed her in this regard, she also came to realize that she did not have to fail herself or her children in the same way. Moving to a new understanding of what it means to be a parent, in light of or in spite of how we were parented, is often a theme in perinatal work.

There are times when client and therapist cry together, and probably as often when the therapist's tears illuminate a feeling or provide a new perspective. Jill described the various roles of tears in our work together in a letter she shared with me regarding tears:

> *About tears in therapy with you and me—it's been there right along, hasn't it? Super important, and also really moving in its own right—it's meant so much to me, but also different things, depending both on when it happened (early in therapy, middle, more recent) and what we were talking about at the time. There were times early on when your tears were this completely illuminating thing, where I was so numb and overwhelmed that I'd just think "Wow . . . I must have said something that's really sad. What was it?" and then I'd think about it and sort of look at it from a distance as this very sad thing that had happened, only just beginning to connect to it. Your tears held it up for me, and not as this awful thing any more—because you were crying over it. Somehow that changed my recognition of it, made it into something loving. Looking at it, wrapping my head around it. Like the tears represented my loving guide—and then I didn't have to sit with just this awful thing and me.*

Jill described my tears as doing more than illuminating a feeling; my tears also reflected a change in her ability to be in touch with her feelings over the course of our work, as well as the changes in her relationship to being helped versus working together. My tears evolved as our work evolved and were a kind of stream through the path of the therapeutic process. As we worked together over several years, Jill looked back down that path and could see what caring looked like, and perhaps could see herself with the grace that was so apparent to me from the beginning.

> *Later on, your tears became something we shared, when I could cry, too, and then they were hugely validating. They let me know I was fully heard, not just in words—like you were there with me, and I knew it from your tears. Over the years, I think we've shifted a bit, where before you were entirely the guide, and now it feels more like moving along this path together, side by side—so the tears now feel a bit different again, like comrades, helpers, people in arms together. Now, after all this time, I think your tears are really all these things at once—it's not like we've gone past the beginning, we've just encompassed more and more.*

Working With Ruth: Tears in the Face of the Unbearable

Ruth[2] was referred to me by a local member of the clergy. Early in our first phone call, she tells me that she has recently been released from prison, and is very grateful for her family's support and the persistent advocacy of her attorney in making this happen. I take a deep breath when this is how a call begins. Hearing me pause, Ruth takes a breath herself and then tells me that she was convicted of manslaughter and incarcerated after the death of her son during a postpartum psychosis. With psychiatric treatment that began in prison, and after her own research, she has come to understand what happened and also realizes that it is highly unusual for her to have been released from prison. She feels both cursed and blessed.

Because I believe it is essential for therapists to use honest observation in our own self-reflection, I notice internally that I have a prejudice: I feel resistant and I feel scared. I don't want to open my heart; it's too hard. *I could refer her on.* The most extreme grief I have experienced as a therapist is while working with mothers who have injured or killed their child during a postpartum psychosis. *Who do I know who could take her?* While I am feeling this resistance, I am also running through a process: *What are the risks? Is this my bias? Does she need help? Do I judge her? Can I handle it?* And again: *Does she need help? Can I provide it?* All of this is going on internally, but I hold steady and keep listening.

As I run through my own process, I am able to assess that Ruth is not psychotic. She is not delusional or hostile, and she is in a world of emotional hurt and grief. For this, I do know how to help her without judgment; in fact, my fears and biases are already starting to recede. Thank goodness for my frequently practiced navigation through my own flight-or-fight reactions. I am still listening, and I make an appointment with her. Suddenly I realize, with sadness and some chagrin, that mothers who have committed what others call "the unthinkable" watch this process occur every time they meet a new person and disclose what happened. Their shame is relentless, their fear and alienation are always with them. And yet, while it may seem contradictory at first, I have learned a great deal about the true depth of maternal love from women who have to survive infanticide committed at their own hands while they were in a temporary psychotic state.

Postpartum psychosis is an illness that is unique to the perinatal time, and if treated appropriately and quickly, is temporary and treatable. Research suggests that psychosis occurs in 1–2 per thousand births, and of that number, a very small percentage complete infanticide, perhaps 4–5% of those who have psychosis (Sit, Rothschild, & Wisner, 2006). Although statistically rare compared to the more common PPD, psychosis is the most extreme and serious perinatal disorder, and requires swift and experienced medical intervention. It is in the recovery and aftermath that psychotherapy enters. Although a rare disorder in the general population, it is not uncommon for experts in perinatal mental health to be called on to counsel women or families who have survived postpartum psychosis, and the smaller number who have experienced the tragedy of infanticide and/or suicide.

When women with postpartum psychosis hurt or kill their children, they are under the influence of uninhibited, irrational, compulsive action driven by delusional beliefs. Women with postpartum psychosis do not hurt or kill their children because they are unhappy mothers, fatigued, or want to remove the child as a barrier. That might sound ridiculous and obvious to a caring reader, and yet all of those derogatory interpretations are used against women accused of crimes during postpartum psychosis. Unlike other psychiatric conditions with chronic and persistent symptoms, postpartum psychosis is temporary and treatable with psychotropic medication and intervention. However, less treatable, and certainly not temporary, are the grief and despair of the mother who is no longer psychotic and has survived her child's injury or death. When I began as a therapist, and before I had experience and knowledge of perinatal mental illness, I could never have imagined the compassion that wells up in me as I sit with the mother who has lost her child to this tragic illness.

Do I cry in the face of that loss? Of course I do. I grieve when I listen to the pain of the mother who was not able find her way without danger. I have cried with families who have lost their daughters and grandchildren, knowing that while my tears accompany their story, they also run the risk of appearing to be a result of shock or judgment. But I understand that for the psychotic woman, the shadow-land of her distorted thoughts became more real and more compelling than any other reality, any other message from her family or moral code. I understand the internal chaos the psychotic woman was living through when she acted on "the unthinkable"; that in the disordered thinking of a postpartum psychosis, she might have believed that it was her imperative as a loving mother to end her child's life so that the baby go directly to heaven or, in some cases, save the world. It is not a rational state of mind. It is not a choice. It is compelled by internal, distorted beliefs. When we have lost such a mother to suicide, or she has ended her child's life, it seems we can only cry, pray, and grieve, and comfort each other.

When Ruth arrives at my office, she is not here to receive treatment for psychosis, or to recover from it. She has been stable for years now. She is here with me to find support for the transition to life after prison, and perhaps the more difficult reality: life after child. She needs to give voice to her immense grief, to find understanding of the illness she experienced, relief from the chronic guilt and depression that remain, and perhaps, if fortunate, a bit of peace and sense of wholeness. I notice my surprise at her gentle appearance, her open and kind face, and her humble approach.

When I suddenly and in person realize how hard it must be for her to come to counseling, I feel my emotion rise and I feel the tears inside, but my professional stance is to keep that private at the beginning. I am still welcoming her. As we get to know one another, and only when I feel confident that she can believe I am not judging or shrinking back in horror, do my tears come to our sessions. When she cries later, I cry with her, and we grieve her loss together. I can never make better what has happened; nobody can fix this. Perhaps this is one of the most important aspects of therapy—working through that which cannot be fixed. When there is no solution to a past tragedy, we can only connect in the shared awareness of pathos, and that is one of the reasons we cry.

CONCLUSION AND RECOMMENDATIONS

Although a psychotherapist who does not specialize in working with the postpartum woman or man might think that study of perinatal mental health is not relevant, remember that prevalence is at least one in seven pregnant or postpartum women and one in ten fathers. The symptoms of pregnancy and postpartum mood and anxiety disorders, childbirth-related trauma, and psychosis are easily misconstrued by providers as having a purely psychodynamic cause. We mistakenly treat the crisis as maternal ambivalence, resistance to the identity of a parent, or even aggression and hostility. Before I became a specialist, it was common for me to exclude intake questions about pregnancy or birth, even if my client had just had a baby. The mental health and medical community have not known enough about perinatal mental health crises, and so we have ignored them at great cost to our clients living with the shame and symptoms of perinatal mood and anxiety disorders, birth trauma, and grief. As with any common but unspoken human experience, when we do not speak of the presence of the common crisis, clients get the message that this is something to be hidden or dealt with as their own failure. Providers must remember that the biggest obstacles to care are the shame and fear a new or expecting parent faces, imagining at worst that the mental health provider will report them as a risk to their child if they disclose how depressed or anxious they are really feeling or if they mention the frightening images that intrude during postpartum obsessive compulsive disorder (Kleiman & Wenzel, 2011).

One of the most poignant moments of counseling perinatal clients, and the time when I most naturally feel my tears, is when I get to tell the new mother that she is not alone, she is not to blame, and that she will get well. I am here to share information with her and to remind her that what she is feeling is not a sign of failure or that she made a mistake trying to or becoming a parent, but that she is living through the symptoms of a temporary, treatable, and understandable response to the biggest transition of her life. I am here to tell her that her suffering is not a sign of failure but a response to a combination of hormonal, social, and psychological vulnerabilities. The reassuring power of psychoeducation in this context can be profound. The mistake that parents and their providers can make, sometimes with tragic consequences, is to view these reactions and symptoms as permanent, a sign of inadequacy or risk to the child, and an inevitable cause of child neglect. We must realize that the greater potential for disrupted attachment comes from the experience of being trapped in this misleading interpretation, mistaking the new mother's symptoms of depression and panic as signs that she should not be with the baby, and that the baby would be better off without her. Far from having a benign effect, the result is that suicide is one of the three leading causes of maternal mortality worldwide (Oates, 2003).

As a therapist and advocate who spends each day supporting women and men coming through this frightening forest of symptoms, what often brings me to tears is to witness vulnerable new parents and would-be parents who are left with these interpretations and, thus, relate to their emerging identity with a sense of failure, despair, and defeat. It is not difficult to reassure them with solid information, to lighten their burden by meeting them with compassion and information about prevalence, resources, and recovery.

I have so often witnessed bonding and attachment truly disrupted not by mental illness or a lack of maternal instinct, but by the vivid fears and shame that have been fertilized in the mind of the parent. When we understand that this new parent is avoiding the child because she mistakenly fears herself and her influence on the child, we suddenly and poignantly see that in fact the protective instinct might be driving the detachment! It has been the greatest surprise of this specialty to observe the potent power of education and reassurance in improving attachment between parent and child. I have cried tears of relief in sessions when observing the scales of fear drop away to reveal the truly nurturing mother or father, and it is always a treasured moment to reflect that back to a new parent. Outside of sessions, I have cried rivers of tears thinking about the global effect and the suffering that could be prevented for new and expecting families if psychoeducation about the emotional vulnerability of new parenthood and an awareness of resources were made available on a broader scale. We have such effective methods and resources to change the intergenerational consequences that are a result more of misinformation than pathology.

In reflecting on my own tears in therapy, there are several important issue that I believe therapists need to keep in mind in working with the perinatal population, as well as any other therapy client.

1. *Remain centered.* It is a commonly accepted standard of psychotherapy that therapists be aware of their own process and remain conscious of projections, conflicts, and reactions that might interfere with the ability to fully perceive and support the client. I experience that process as a centering, and that ability to find my center in sessions requires ongoing self-care in my daily life and consistent attentiveness in client interactions. How do we remain responsive but able to touch and find our center at any moment? Therapists need to be able to ride the wave of emotions but not create waves from their own reactions. We need to respond to the shifts of feeling, but always be able to return to center so that we are more responsive to clients than to our own needs. I have learned to allow my spontaneous tears as a therapist, but also to be mindful of when they are more of a distraction to the client's process. I have to be very present, watch for even the slightest pulling back or evidence that I am distracting my client, and stop my tears.

2. *Respect your client's interpersonal space.* We also need to respect where we are in the process of getting to know one another, and be aware of the emotional climate generated by the client in the session. *I follow my client's level of comfort with emotion to guide the expression of my own.* The appropriateness of the therapist's tears changes over the course of therapy as we get to know one another and develop trust and timing. If that is respected, the therapist illustrates the interpersonal boundaries that respond to the client's changing needs for intimacy and individuation. When the timing of interpersonal intimacy feels safe, the compassionate response of tears can remind and illustrate to clients a natural compassion for themselves and a lifting of the burden of shame and self-recrimination.

One of the most important tasks of the perinatal therapist is to guide and teach the new mother and father to be a safe person for their child, to hold an empathic and consistent space for the baby in need of attachment. In wordless ways, we practice this experience in therapy, sharing with our clients the neurobiology of attachment, which is often accompanied by the sharing of tears as well as humor (Siegel & Hartzell, 2004). I believe that children of healthy mothers are accustomed to seeing their mothers cry. Mothers are notorious for crying over their children's heartbreak but also over their joys. The same process exists in therapy. A caring therapist might naturally cry when witnessing the heartbreak of the client, but also when there is a newfound joy, or relief that springs up with new growth. Working with families in this immensely vulnerable time of life, I often find tears on my face when we have realized together that the storm has passed; there is freedom from shame, and compassion for the pain that she stumbled through along the path to recovery. I will sometimes see the baby years later, a grown-up adolescent or teen, and marvel again at the miracle of healing and recovery. What an honor to walk along that path for a while with a client, during the birth of a new parent. For it is indeed a birth, and for most of us it is inevitable to cry at a birth. We are forever moved by the Herculean effort of the mother, the innocence of the baby's need for comfort, the pain that has passed, the risk of danger averted, and the everlasting potential for life to emerge protected and whole.

NOTES

1. Biographical information and case details have been changed to protect the identity of clients.
2. Biographical information and case details have been changed to protect the identity of clients.

REFERENCES

Brealey, S. D., Hewitt, C., Green, J. M., Morrell, J., & Gilbody, S. (2010). Screening for postnatal depression—is it acceptable to women and healthcare professionals? A systematic review and meta-synthesis. *Journal of Reproductive and Infant Psychology, 28*(4), 328–344.

Eaton, N. R., Keyes, K. M., Krueger, R. F., Balsis, S., Skodol, A. E., Markon, K. E., . . . Hasin, D. S. (2012). An invariant dimensional liability model of gender differences in mental disorder prevalence: Evidence from a national sample. *Journal of Abnormal Psychology, 121*(2), 282–288.

Kleiman, K., & Wenzel, A. (2011). *Dropping the baby and other scary thoughts: Breaking the cycle of unwanted thoughts in motherhood.* New York, NY: Routledge.

Meltzer-Brody, S. (2011). New insights into perinatal depression: Pathogenesis and treatment during pregnancy and postpartum. *Dialogues in Clinical Neuroscience, 13*(1), 89–100.

Oates, M. (2003). Suicide: The leading cause of maternal death. *British Journal of Psychiatry, 183*(4), 279–281.

Paulson, J. F., & Bazemore, S. D. (2010). Prenatal and postpartum depression in fathers and its association with maternal depression: A meta-analysis. *JAMA, 303*(19), 1961–1969.

Siegel, D. J., & Hartzell, M. (2004). *Parenting from the inside out: How a deeper self-understanding can help you raise children who thrive.* New York, NY: J.P. Tarcher/Penguin.

Sit, D., Rothschild, A. J., & Wisner, K. L. (2006). A review of postpartum psychosis. *Journal of Women's Health, 15*(4), 352–368.

Vingerhoets, A. J. J. M., & Bylsma, L. M. (2015). The riddle of human emotional crying: A challenge for emotion researchers. *Emotion Review,* 1–11.

Wisner, K. L., Sit, D. K. Y., McShea, M. C., Rizzo, D. M., Zoretich, R. A., Hughes, C. L., . . . Hanusa, B. H. (2013). Onset timing, thoughts of self-harm, and diagnoses in postpartum women with screen-positive depression findings. *JAMA Psychiatry, 70*(5), 490–498.

CHAPTER 14

SUPERVISING OUR TEARS: A GUIDE FOR SUPERVISORS AND TRAINEES

Amy Blume-Marcovici, Kelsey E. Schraufnagel, Mojgan Khademi, and Ronald A. Stolberg

I (AB) was a practicum student at an outpatient mental health clinic, when I first met Derek.[1] He had been referred for depression secondary to a car accident that left him paralyzed from the waist down, with pain in the parts of his body he could no longer move or otherwise feel. As we settled into my office for his intake appointment, I was struck by how withdrawn Derek seemed. He was 35 years old and he sat hunched over in his wheelchair, with his head hung low, barely making eye contact. His voice was so quiet that my own seemed to boom, despite my attempts to lower my volume to match his. When he spoke, it was with an apologetic tone, as if he felt even his thoughts were a burden.

It was not until our eighth meeting that Derek told me the full story of the car accident five years prior which resulted in his paralysis and subsequent pain: he had been rushing to his mother's house after she had threatened to commit suicide. I learned that there was a long history of such threats, often following something positive in Derek's life, such as a new friend or school interest, which might require him to spend time away from home. Whenever his mother told Derek of

(continued)

(continued)

her intention to kill herself, Derek rushed home and would not leave the house for days, sometimes weeks. On the day of the accident—a week after Derek's wedding—Derek was rushing to his mother's home believing that she had taken a bottle of pills. Derek did not remember anything after getting into the car, but he was told that he had barreled through a red light, was hit by another car, and was "lucky" to be alive.

As Derek described the accident, his face and tone devoid of emotion or inflection, I felt my eyes well up with tears and a few spill on to my cheeks. I saw that Derek noticed my tears, but did not comment on them. Nor did I. I felt instantly distracted: pulled away from Derek's experience and consumed by worry that I had committed an unspoken professional breach. I was relieved that Derek continued talking, in his familiar monotone whisper, and that he confirmed our next appointment before he left.

There I sat in my office, feeling terribly confused by what had happened. I had felt so connected with Derek and honored that he had shared a story he had rarely spoken aloud. I also felt deeply concerned I had burdened him—a man who already felt like a burden, emotionally and physically, to everyone in his life—with my own tears. I worried that he would question whether he could trust me to endure his pain. I was also caught off guard. Why had I cried? Why now? Why with Derek?

In retrospect, I am surprised that I was so surprised by my tears. I am a crier, I always have been. Even a good commercial can have me weeping. But somehow I never thought about how my tears might show up in my new role as a therapist. Quite honestly, if naively, I assumed they would not. And then, all of the sudden, there I was, crying with a client! My clinical supervision at the time focused on working with clients with different abilities, and we discussed the emotional intensity of working with a client who was paralyzed and severely depressed. And yet, still, I was embarrassed by my own emotionality and concerned about the impact this had on Derek and our relationship. In addition, I felt doubly ashamed because not only had I cried, but I had not had the professional wherewithal to handle it in the way I was sure a "good" therapist would have.

Despite my embarrassment, I presented Derek's case—and my tears—to my consultation group, as I knew I needed support and guidance. In preparing my presentation, I found a beautiful article, written by psychologist Caroline Owens

(2005), on the subject of therapist tears (one of three existing case studies related to this topic at that time); lo and behold, she wrote about crying with a client who was paralyzed and many of the themes she discussed resonated with my work with Derek. She discussed the role of projection and projective identification, the defense processes through which her quadriplegic 13-year-old client mobilized the people in his life around him, and ultimately moved her to cry tears that she believed were his. In other words, she cried his tears just as others in his life helped him perform basic functions that his paralysis left him unable to perform. Owens' conceptualization of tears as a form of movement in the room somehow normalized and clarified my tears for me, and this idea became the basis for my discussion with my consultation group and an important theme in my work with Derek. We discussed the ways in which Derek felt "stuck": stuck in the pain he experienced in the parts of his body he could not move, stuck to relive his mother's depression and hopelessness, stuck in his wheelchair, which brought up similar feelings for Derek as when he had felt stuck in his house during his mother's "episodes." What we learned was that, while Derek was "stuck" with physical limitations, we could work to help him become "unstuck" emotionally, and this might ultimately provide him with a sense of freedom. Indeed, emotions—a word that has its etymology in the Latin term emovere, which means "to move"—was the key way in which movement, and progress, occurred in our work. In one of the more poignant illustrations of this, Derek shared with me that he was feeling suicidal. He disclosed that he struggled with such feelings frequently, but had never told anyone for fear of being like his own mother. In trusting me with these thoughts and feelings, Derek himself began to cry, the first time he had done so since his accident.

I am still not sure how Derek interpreted or felt about my tears, as I never asked him. I wonder if he felt burdened by them; or if my tears helped him feel a connection to me that eventually allowed him to have his own tears. Perhaps both are true. Regardless, because of what I learned upon reflection, reading, and consultation about my tears, I was able to use this experience to deepen our work. In fact, had I not cried, my work with Derek may not have taken on the important themes that it did. In presenting Derek's case to my consultation group, I found a supportive community who—though ranging considerably in their reactions to the idea of therapists' tears—helped me think through the potential detrimental and constructive aspects of my tears. It is from this experience—my positive experience of consultation around tears and my experience in the room with Derek—and my subsequent belief that exploration, understanding, and attention to moments of tearfulness are beneficial, that this chapter (and indeed this whole book) springs forth.

The majority of psychologists cry in therapy (Blume-Marcovici, Stolberg, & Khademi, 2013; Brownlie, 2014; Pope, Tabachnick, & Keith-Spiegel, 1987; 't Lam & Vingerhoets, 2016; Tritt, Kelly, & Waller, 2015). However, the majority of therapists do not discuss their experience of crying with clients in supervision or trainings, despite the fact that therapists almost unanimously believe that they should receive training on how to handle their own emotions in therapy sessions (Blume-Marcovici, Stolberg, Khademi, & Giromini, 2015; 't Lam & Vingerhoets, 2016). In this chapter, we describe the current state of research as it relates to training and supervision on therapist crying as well as provide training and supervision guidelines and sample exercises to address therapists' tears.

RESEARCH ON SUPERVISION AND TRAINING IN REGARD TO THERAPISTS' CRYING

Only two empirical studies have focused on supervision and training in regard to therapist tearfulness. One, by 't Lam and Vingerhoets (2016), found that approximately 61% of the 819 mental health workers who responded to their survey on therapist crying felt there was not enough attention paid to the topic of therapists' tears in their training, while almost all (92%) felt that it was necessary to address therapists' emotional expressions, including crying. The other study, by Blume-Marcovici et al. (2015), found that the majority of the 684 psychologists and psychology trainees who took part in their study reported that the subject of therapists' tears was not broached in a formal way during the entirety of their training. Approximately half of these respondents reported discussing their tears in therapy with their supervisor, while one-quarter never disclosed the act of crying in therapy to anyone. While a little more than half of the survey participants appeared to feel prepared to handle their crying in therapy, over a quarter reported that they did not. Notably, this study found that having received focused training on therapists' tears in therapy correlated with feeling more prepared to handle tears when they happened. The less prepared the therapist, the more he or she tended to report regretting having cried, both in the form of wishing he or she had not cried as well as feeling that crying represented a therapeutic mistake.

Male therapists reported significantly fewer experiences of training and supervision on therapists' tears and were less likely to discuss their own tears with a supervisor or colleague than their female counterparts, *despite equal rates of crying in therapy* amongst men and women (Blume-Marcovici et al., 2013). Researchers have found men to have more negative feelings about their own sex's tears than about females' tears (Lombardo, Cretser, Lombardo, & Mathis, 1983). Thus, it is possible that male therapists feel ashamed or are concerned that their tears violate important gender norms regarding emotional expression (Levant, 2001) and thus avoid discussing tears with a supervisor. Additionally, these same biases around emotional expression and gender may decrease supervisors' likelihood to inquire about their male trainees' emotional expression and tears.

Dynamically oriented therapists tend to report more supervision focused on their tears and how to handle them than cognitive-behavioral therapists, despite the vast majority of both groups reporting that training on the subject is important (Blume-Marcovici et al., 2013). The reason for the differences in supervision and training experiences between these two groups may be explained in part by the emphasis placed on emotional expression within the psychodynamic framework as compared to other orientations (Blagys & Hilsenroth, 2000); this likely carries over into the supervision and training process.

Although therapist crying may be perceived differently by the various theoretical frameworks, with some models finding therapist tearfulness to be functionally beneficial with a particular client and others discouraging it altogether, research suggests that such emotional expression occurs for therapists across all modalities. As such, it is our belief that any model of supervision, regardless of the particular orientation of the therapist, would do well to address therapist tearfulness with trainees. In fact, some treatment models already do so. For instance, functional analytic psychotherapy (Kohlenberg & Tsai, 1991), an interpersonal, contextual, and behavioral therapy that emphasizes the therapeutic relationship and in-session interactions to shape clients' interpersonal behaviors and promote meaningful and satisfying relationships, addresses the topic of therapist emotional expression, including therapist crying, in its intensive trainings (Kohlenberg, 2015) and supervision (Tsai et al., 2008). Below, we provide transtheoretical guidelines and exercises to encourage discussion and exploration of therapists' tears in supervision and training settings. We encourage adapting the exercises as necessary to fit the setting and time availability.

TEARS IN SUPERVISION AND TRAINING: RECOMMENDATIONS AND TRAINING EXERCISES

Guidelines for Discussion of Therapist Tearfulness[2]

- *Supervisory alliance.* A supportive supervisory relationship is imperative for creating a foundation from which to discuss sensitive experience(s), such as therapist crying. It is important that supervisors prioritize a strong working alliance, which can be established through collaboratively setting supervision goals and creating a strong emotional bond (Bordin, 1994).

- *Normalize.* The majority of therapists have experienced tears in therapy with a client at some point in their career, with estimates ranging from 57% (Tritt et al., 2015) to 87% ('t Lam & Vingerhoets, 2016). A supervisor can help to reduce potential feelings of discomfort, shame, or regret through normalization (Hahn, 2001). In fact, we suggest pre-emptive normalization by helping trainees anticipate and prepare for tears in therapy (see training exercises below).
- *Supervisor self-disclosure of tears in therapy.* Supervisors may consider sharing their own experience(s) of tearfulness in therapy with their supervisee, particularly when the supervisor determines that: (1) such sharing may help normalize a supervisee's experience; and (2) such sharing may strengthen the supervisory working alliance and increase the likelihood of supervisee disclosure.
- *Men cry, too.* While male and female therapists report similar rates of crying in therapy, male trainees are significantly less likely to seek supervision regarding their tears. Thus, supervisors may need to be proactive in asking about, normalizing, or eliciting discussion of tears with male trainees. Similarly, since research has found tearfulness to occur at equal rates amongst all ethnic groups (Blume-Marcovici et al., 2015), supervisors should be aware of any biases or cultural stereotypes regarding emotional expression that might make a supervisee less likely to disclose tears or make the supervisor less likely to broach the topic.
- *Hot topics.* The most common session topics during which therapists report crying are grief, trauma, and termination (Blume-Marcovici, Stolberg, & Khademi, 2015); forced termination was particularly likely to be accompanied by tears. Because forced terminations are a common reality for many trainees (due to year-long training placements that often result in concluding with a client prior to treatment goals being met), it may be particularly helpful to pre-emptively discuss therapists' emotional expressions and tears in anticipation of and during these transitions and endings.
- *Mixed emotions.* Research shows that, when therapists cry, they often feel a combination of emotions, both positive and negative, such as sadness *and* warmth toward a client (Blume-Marcovici et al., 2013). In fact, some research finds that emotions tend to be more positive than negative in these tearful moments (Brownlie, 2014). Supervisors can help supervisees to understand their own range of emotional response when tears occur in

order to deepen their understanding of the complex emotional exchange between therapist/trainee and client.

- *Discussion of therapist's tears with the client.* When a therapist cries in therapy, should the incident be discussed with the client? Research shows a correlation between discussing therapists' tears with clients and increased rapport (Blume-Marcovici et al., 2015). Supervisors can support supervisees in considering both the process and implications of such a discussion, including how to broach the topic with a particular client after the therapist cried with the client or, more generally, in anticipating how the therapist might address his/her tears in future sessions or potential experiences with therapist tears in therapy.
- *Parallel process.* If therapists sometimes cry in therapy, surely supervisors also tear up, at times, in supervision. Discussion of supervisor emotionality during supervision might lead to a discovery of parallels between the supervisory and therapy process (Searles, 1955). Perhaps the supervisor's tears reflect emotions felt by the therapist/trainee and/or client. Discussion of the supervisor's emotionality might also create opportunities for metacommunication about the supervisory relationship that could enhance supervisee communication with his or her own clients (Tracey, Bludworth, & Glidden-Tracey, 2011). Indeed, permission from the supervisor to discuss this often undiscussed topic in supervision might provide trainees with a model for discussing tears in therapy with their own clients.

Training Exercises

We have developed a three-part training exercise to serve as a framework for facilitating reflection and learning about the topic of therapists' crying in therapy. *Part 1: Understanding Our Tears* focuses on helping therapists formulate their beliefs about crying and understand their own relationship to tears. *Part II: Working with the Crying Client* emphasizes understanding the therapist's thoughts and feelings about clients' crying. *Part III: Working with Therapists' Tears* focuses on therapists' tears in therapy. Each section includes an experiential exercise to facilitate a deep level of reflection, followed by discussion questions. The exercise can be offered as a group training, incorporated into clinical supervision, or conducted independently as a self-reflection activity. We recommend that the three-part exercise be conducted over an extended training or supervision session (ideally approximately 90 minutes, with 30 minutes devoted to each section). If less time is available, supervisors can choose one of the sections and use the exercise and discussion in that section for a 30–45-minute training. For each section of the training, we have included transcripts of the experiential exercises. If you choose to conduct this exercise as an independent, self-reflection activity, we encourage you to audio-record yourself reading the transcripts and play them back at a pace that feels right for you. Journaling your thoughts and feelings about each of the discussion questions might also deepen your experience.

INTRODUCTION

We recommend spending five to ten minutes at the beginning of the session to introduce the topic of crying and set the stage for this training exercise. We have included an outline of an introduction below, but we encourage facilitators to personalize it. For instance, you could formulate questions based on the research presented to encourage participation. Of import, because of the personal and sensitive nature of the topic—crying—if the facilitator does not know the trainees already, we encourage taking time to develop rapport at the start.

> *Transcript*
>
> *Today we are going to be discussing an important topic that we often do not directly talk about in our culture, or even in psychotherapy training: crying. We'll begin by examining our own relationship to crying, then move on to discuss client crying, and finally talk about therapists' crying in therapy. Given that crying is such a personal and intimate experience, it makes sense if you feel uncomfortable or anxious. I want to encourage you to be curious and open, as much as you are willing, as we reflect on crying in various contexts.*
>
> *Now, I would like to start by asking you to silently reflect on a few questions. First, how many times have you cried in the last month, if at all? (Pause) Do you consider yourself a crier? Have others labeled you as such? Or are you someone who "never cries"? (Pause). Do you believe there is value in crying? What about in the therapy setting; is it important for clients to cry in therapy? (Pause) Is it ever okay for the therapist to cry in a session?*
>
> (Below we have included research bullet points on crying; you are welcome to share any or all of this information as part of your introduction to the exercises. If you are less familiar with the group, more time on this didactic component at the start may help to establish rapport and comfort.)

I'm now going to talk for a moment about what research tells us about crying, both in general and in therapy, and then we'll move on to to the more experiential aspects of this training.

- *Research worldwide finds that women cry more than men. In the United States, adult women tend to cry two to five times a month, whereas adult men report crying once every two months (Vingerhoets & Bylsma, 2015).*
- *Our current understanding of crying has focused on crying as an attachment behavior. From this perspective, crying is an inborn, universal behavior present from birth that serves to beckon the caregiver when the infant is in need of help and care. Adult crying is seen as a continuation of this attachment behavior, reflective of our caregiving needs and attempts at soliciting a caregiver (Nelson, 2005).*
- *In therapy, clients cry on average once out of every seven sessions (Robinson, Hill, & Kivighan, 2015).*
- *Some research has looked at attachment theory in regard to crying in therapy, and has shown that client crying in therapy is associated with the client's attachment style (Nelson, 2005; Robinson et al., 2015), as well as the attachment style of the therapist (Robinson et al., 2015). For instance, when therapists have an avoidant attachment style, their clients tend to cry more at the beginning of therapy, but less over time. When therapists have an anxious attachment style, clients tend to exhibit more protest—or angry—crying. Therapists who establish a secure attachment have clients who cry more overall.*
- *Despite the fact that clients tend to describe therapy sessions in which they cry as more difficult than others, they describe the therapeutic alliance as strong in these sessions (Capps, Fiori, Mullin, & Hilsenroth, 2015).*
- *Not only the client cries in therapy. Research has shown that the majority of therapists have experienced their own tears in therapy, with estimates ranging from 57% (Brownlie, 2014) to 87% ('t Lam & Vingerhoets, 2016). Most of the time, therapists report having "tears in their eyes" as opposed to more intense crying, though more intense crying does also occur.*
- *Research suggests that therapists who identify as "criers" in their daily life, outside of therapy, are more likely to cry in therapy. Research also shows that therapists with more clinical experience tend to cry more frequently in therapy. Interestingly, male and female therapists report equal rates of crying in therapy, even when these same respondents report the typical sex differences of crying in daily life (i.e., female therapists cry more than male therapists in daily life).*

PART 1: UNDERSTANDING OUR TEARS

As a first step, it is important to increase participants' awareness and understanding of their own tears, which can be encouraged through reflection on opinions about, and personal experiences with, crying. The experiential practices in this section may evoke strong or uncomfortable emotions for participants. We suggest that facilitators try to balance encouraging participants' vulnerability and openness, while respecting their personal boundaries and comfort levels. It may also be helpful to provide options for additional support following the exercises as necessary.

Experiential Exercise: Your Tears

Transcript

I'd now like to invite you to participate in an experiential exercise. To begin this exercise, I'd like to ask everyone to put down anything you might be holding and find a centered and balanced position in your chair (model upright positioning and then pause). *Perhaps close your eyes if that feels comfortable for you; otherwise you can narrow and soften your gaze just a few feet in front of you.*

And now take a few deep breaths; inhaling all the way down into your lower abdomen, before exhaling slowly and completely. (Pause)

Now, with your eyes closed or looking downward, I am going to ask a few questions that I would like you to silently reflect upon.

What words or images come to mind when you think about crying? (Pause)

Notice any sensations in your body as you consider these words and images. (Pause)

Now, take a few moments to try and recall a time when you have cried. (Pause) *This may be a time from your childhood, or perhaps more recent.* (Pause)

It may be a particularly memorable experience, or the first memory that came to mind. (Pause)

You might have cried intensely or for a long time, or perhaps you simply teared up. (Pause for about 30 seconds)

Now, while your eyes are still closed or looking downward, I'm going to ask you a few questions about this experience for you to reflect on.

> *What caused you to tear up or cry in this situation?* (Pause)
>
> *How were you feeling at the time?* (Pause)
>
> *Were you with someone or were you alone?* (Pause)
>
> *What was your reaction to your tears? Did you try to stop them? Or did you let your tears flow freely?* (Pause)
>
> *Did anyone say anything to you about your tears?* (Pause)
>
> *How did your feelings change after you cried?* (Give trainees a few extra moments here)
>
> *Finally, take a moment to reflect on how you feel right now, having just thought back on this experience. Are the emotions similar or different to those you felt in that moment?* (Pause)
>
> *What sensations do you notice in your body now?* (Pause)
>
> *Is there a desire to have this exercise end, to be alone, or maybe to share or process your experience?* (Pause)
>
> *Take a slow, deep breath, and when you are ready, please slowly open your eyes.* (Pause)

Discussion: Your Tears

Below we have provided questions to facilitate a discussion around the participants' experience of crying.

1. What was your experience doing this exercise? Was it difficult to recall a memory or hard to choose between memories? How was it to think back on your moment? Did you notice similar feelings arise now as were present in your moment? Or different?
2. When you think of crying, what images or ideas come to mind?
3. What has shaped your opinions about crying? Do you have any recollections from your childhood of messages you were given about crying? Has your opinion of crying, yours or others', changed over the years?
4. Think back to the question I asked you at the start of our discussion: Are you "a crier"? What causes a person to be "a crier"? What leads a person to "never cry"? How do you think your gender has affected your feelings about crying?

5. As you reflect on your experiences of crying—both the one that you just focused on, and also more generally—do you notice whether you are more likely to cry in "positive" emotional (e.g., joy, sentimentality) or "negative" emotional (e.g., sad, angry) situations? Both? Neither? Do you feel differently about crying based on the emotional context? (Note to facilitator: research shows that men report crying more due to "positive" emotional situations whereas women tend to report crying more due to "negative" emotional situations; Vingerhoets & Bylsma, 2015.)

PART II: WORKING WITH THE CRYING CLIENT

This portion of the training aims to increase participants' awareness of their own feelings about and reactions to other people's tears, and how this impacts their experience of clients' tears.

Experiential Exercise: Being With Tears

Transcript

Please take a moment to settle back into your chair and close your eyes or look downward, softening your gaze. (Pause)

Take a few slow, deep breaths, preparing again to engage in some reflection. (Pause)

I'd like you to now think of a time when you were with a client who cried. (Pause 30 seconds)

What was happening in the room when this client started to cry?

Take a moment to picture the face of this client, as they were crying. (Pause)

Did they have tears coming down their cheeks? Did they use a Kleenex to wipe their tears or allow their tears to flow?

What was their body posture? (Pause)

Were they looking at you? Away from you? (Pause)

Did their crying make any noise? (Pause)

> *Did they seem comfortable with their tears, or try to stop them? Did they apologize for their tears?* (Pause)
>
> *What do you believe they were feeling?* (Pause)
>
> *Take another slow, deep breath and shift your focus to what you were feeling.* (Pause)
>
> *What emotions do you remember feeling in that moment?* (Pause)
>
> *What thoughts went through your mind?* (Pause)
>
> *Do you remember being aware of any sensations in your body?* (Pause)
>
> *Do you notice any sensations in your body now, as you think back to this experience?* (Pause)
>
> *What did you feel toward your client as they cried?* (Pause)
>
> *What did you have an urge to do in that moment?* (Pause)
>
> *What did you actually do, if anything? Did you move your body toward them? Look or move away? Did you say anything?* (Pause)
>
> *Did you have any impulse to cry yourself? Did you have tears in your eyes?* (Pause) *If so, how did that feel?*
>
> *When you are ready, take a deep breath and open your eyes.*

Discussion: Being With Tears

Ask trainees to reflect on the above exercise as you discuss the following questions.

1. What was it like to do that exercise? Was it easy or difficult to recall, or to choose, a specific instance? Would anyone like to share their experience of a client crying?
2. Do you think it is helpful for clients to cry in therapy? Why or why not?
3. What should the role of the therapist be when a client cries?
4. Does the gender of the client influence your reaction to the client's tears? How many of you recalled a female client in this exercise? How many of you recalled a male client? How might the gender of the therapist influence the client's experience of his or her own tears?

5. Have you ever had a time when you felt uncomfortable in any way in the face of your client's tears (e.g., annoyed, helpless, frustrated, angry)?
6. How do you think your own early experiences with crying, as well as your feelings about your own tears, impact your reaction to your clients' crying?

PART III: WORKING WITH THERAPISTS' TEARS IN THERAPY

This final portion of the training focuses on therapists' tears in therapy by specifically evoking beliefs about and experiences with therapists' tears in therapy. In this portion of the training, the facilitator should reflect upon whether he/she has an experience of tears in therapy him/herself that might be shared with the group to inspire discussion, if you find that the group is hesitant to share experiences at first.

Experiential Exercise: Therapists' Tears

Transcript

Take a moment to get comfortable in your chair. Begin to soften your gaze and, if you're comfortable, close your eyes. (Pause)

Think of a time when you have teared up or cried with a client in your role as a therapist. (Pause)

If you have not experienced this, reflect on whether you own therapist ever teared up or cried during therapy with you. If you have not experienced either of these, think back to a time when you may have felt an intense emotion with a client, perhaps a time when you wondered or worried that these feelings may have shown to your client.

Focus your awareness on what was happening in the therapy room when you teared up or cried—or felt an intense emotion that you thought your client may have noticed.

Who was your client? (Pause)

What were you, or your client, discussing at the time? (Pause)

> *At what point in treatment did your crying occur? Intake session or termination? Early or late in treatment?* (Pause)
>
> *What were you feeling when you cried?* (Pause)
>
> *Did you do or say anything in relation to your tears? Did you attempt to blink or wipe away your tears? Perhaps let them come?* (Pause)
>
> *What do you believe your client was feeling at the time you teared up?* (Pause)
>
> *Was your client crying? Did your client notice your tears?* (Pause)
>
> *Did you discuss your tears with your client?* (Pause)
>
> *How do you think your crying impacted the therapy?* (Pause)
>
> *When you are ready, open your eyes.*

Discussion: Therapists' Tears

Ask trainees to reflect on the above exercise as you discuss the following questions.

1. How many of you recalled a time when you have teared up or cried in therapy? How was it for you to think back on this moment? Would anyone be willing to share their experience?
2. Did anyone use this exercise to reflect on a time that their own therapist teared up or cried in therapy, or when you may have felt an intense emotion with a client that you thought your client may have noticed? Would anyone be willing to share that experience?
3. Why might therapists cry in therapy? Are some therapists more likely to cry than others?
4. What are the possible positive effects of therapists' tears? In what scenarios can you imagine these to occur?
5. What are the possible negative effects of therapists' tears? In what scenarios can you imagine these to occur? Are there certain clients with whom you feel therapists should never cry?
6. How should therapists handle crying in therapy? Do you think therapists should discuss their own tears with their client? In which situations?
7. Does crying differ from other emotional expression? Laughing? Getting angry?

SUMMARY AND GUIDELINES

The conclusion of this training segues from Part III and focuses specifically on guidelines and suggestions for trainees regarding how to manage tears in therapy, as we have found trainees often crave such a discussion. Feel free to use some or all of these points as you provide this information to trainees.

> *Transcript*
>
> - *Research shows that when a therapist talks about his or her tears with a client, the therapist reports his or her tears to have a positive impact on the therapy more often than a neutral or negative impact (Blume-Marcovici et al., 2015). Research on clients' perception of their therapist's tears suggests a more complex story, with clients having a stronger response (positive or negative) to therapists' not discussing their tears. Specifically, when clients have a negative response to a therapist's tears, they describe feeling responsible or burdened by the tears, sometimes leading the client to end therapy; alternatively, when clients report a positive response to their therapist's tears, they describe feeling that their therapist's tears expressed more than words could say and appreciated silence and space around tears (Watson, 2015). However, since clients do not tend to report a negative reaction to therapists' discussing tears, when in doubt about the potential impact of tears on a client, finding a client-centered way to discuss the therapist's tears is good practice. I'm going to discuss a few general guidelines about how to effectively discuss therapist tears with clients, keeping in mind, however, that consideration of the unique therapist–client dyad is most important in determining the best course of action.*
>   - *Discussion of tears can be as brief as an acknowledgment of the therapist's feelings that arose while listening to or empathizing with the client's experience (i.e., "I am feeling deeply moved as I listen to you talk about this"). Alternatively, the discussion may be more in depth, such as when the therapist or client has an interpretation about the unique meaning of the therapist's tears to the client (e.g., tearing up when working with a client who is devoid of any emotion, or with a client who tends to avoid interpersonal intimacy), and a discussion around the interpersonal aspect of tears may lead to insight for the client, or provide the client with the type of intimate or vulnerable interpersonal exchange that he/she may be struggling to manifest in life outside of therapy.*
>   - *Discussing tears does not need to happen as tears are occurring. In fact, this may detract from the moment, especially if tears occur in the midst of an intense emotional response for the client. In this case, it may be more beneficial to discuss the therapist's response later in the session or to revisit it at the following session.*

- *It is very important to keep a client-centered perspective when discussing therapists' tears. If a therapist's tears are in response to her or his own personal struggles, a brief acknowledgment of the therapist's emotional state might suffice. The therapist should think carefully about what and how much to disclose in such instances, and certainly should be prepared to help the client process the therapist's tears should they be perceived as intruding on the client's space.*
- *Note that crying in response to one's own personal struggles during therapy (which therapists report happens quite rarely) is qualitatively different than an empathic response to a client's experience which might be heightened by a resonance with the therapist's similar personal experience (which is more commonly reported). Acknowledgment of such resonance may or may not be helpful; focusing on the strong empathic connection and using this to deepen one's understanding of the client's experience is most important.*

- *If a therapist determines that his/her tears were not appropriate or useful, and worries that he/she is prone to tears again with this client, it may be helpful to seek consultation and/or talk with one's own therapist in order to process relevant emotions or events that are affecting the therapist's work. It might also be particularly useful for those therapists who are "criers" in daily life to learn and develop strategies for managing strong emotional responses (e.g., brief mindfulness of breath practice before the session and/or during the session). If a therapist finds him- or herself crying very often in therapy sessions, it may be important to do some personal reflection on the experience, as frequent crying is outside the norm of most therapists' experience. Note that there is an argument to be made that suppressing one's emotional response, such as tears, is inauthentic and that there may be useful information in such responses that would be lost due to suppression. The balance between authenticity and protecting the space for the client is a careful and essential one to strike. If a therapist feels the urge to tear up in a session but feels it would be distracting, unhelpful, or harmful to the client, try to postpone your tears, but allow them to come later. In allowing your tears at another time, you might learn something about the client, or yourself, that was missing in the session.*
- *Above all else, it feels important to reiterate that most therapists do experience tearfulness in therapy at some point. Even when a client experiences a therapist's tears as a rupture in the alliance, with attunement by the therapist to the unique reaction of the client, and an appropriate client-centered therapeutic response, such ruptures can be repaired. Certainly not all therapists' tears are experienced as a rupture, and in fact, tears in and of themselves can be perceived by clients as a connected, attuned, and appropriate caregiving response.*

CONCLUSION

In this chapter, we have discussed the pertinent research in relation to supervision and training on therapists' tears in therapy. As we have shown, the research base is small, and discussion of this topic is very new to the psychotherapy literature. Using the available research as a foundation, we have developed guidelines for supervisors working with supervisees, which we presented in the section, "Guidelines for Discussion of Therapist Tearfulness," as well as a small-group style training, outlined above, on crying in therapy. Future research on the topic of supervising trainees in relation to crying in general (their own and their clients'), as well as other emotional expressions, is essential in the effort to develop effective, evidence-based guidelines regarding therapist emotional expression in therapy.

NOTES

1. In this vignette, I have attempted to capture the emotional truth about my (AB's) experience of crying in therapy with a client when I was a trainee. In order to maintain the client's anonymity, the case description I provided is an amalgam of various cases with many fictionalized details, such that it does not represent any real client.
2. Several of these guidelines are also discussed in Blume-Marcovici et al. (2015).

REFERENCES

Blagys, M. D., & Hilsenroth, M. J. (2000). Distinctive features of short-term psychodynamic-interpersonal psychotherapy: A review of the comparative psychotherapy process literature. *Clinical Psychology: Science and Practice, 7*, 167–188.

Blume-Marcovici, A. C., Stolberg, R. A., & Khademi, M. (2013). Do therapists cry in therapy? The role of experience and other factors in therapists' tears. *Psychotherapy: Theory, Research, Practice, Training, 50*(2), 224–234.

Blume-Marcovici, A. C., Stolberg, R. A., & Khademi, M. (2015). Examining our tears: Therapists' accounts of crying in therapy. *American Journal of Psychotherapy, 69*(4), 399–421.

Blume-Marcovici, A. C., Stolberg, R. A., Khademi, K., & Giromini, L. (2015). When therapists cry: Implications for supervision and training. *The Clinical Supervisor, 34*(2), 164–183.

Bordin, E. S. (1994). Theory and research in the therapeutic working alliance: New directions. In A. O. Horvath & L. S. Greenberg (Eds.), *The working alliance: Theory, research and practice* (pp. 13–37). New York, NY: Wiley.

Brownlie, M. R. (2014). *Uncharted 'tearitory': Mapping Australian therapist experiences, attitudes, and understandings of their in-session tears.* Unpublished master's thesis. Monash University, Australia.

Capps, K. L., Fiori, K., Mullin, A. S., & Hilsenroth, M. J. (2015). Patient crying in psychotherapy: Who cries and why? *Clinical Psychology and Psychotherapy, 22*(3), 208–220.

Hahn, W. K. (2001). The experience of shame in psychotherapy supervision. *Psychotherapy, 38*, 272–282.

Kohlenberg, B. (2015, May). Rules, relational framing, and augmentals. *Functional Analytic Psychotherapy Intensive.* Symposium conducted at the meeting of University of Washington, Seattle.

Kohlenberg, R. J., & Tsai, M. (1991) *Functional analytic psychotherapy: Creating intense and curative therapeutic relationships.* New York, NY: Plenum.

Levant, R. F. (2001). Desperately seeking language: Understanding, assessing, and treating normative male alexithymia. In G. R. Brooks & G. E. Good (Eds.), *The new handbook of psychotherapy and counseling with men: A comprehensive guide to settings, problems, and treatment approaches* (Vols. 1 & 2, pp. 424–443). San Francisco, CA: Jossey-Bass.

Lombardo, W. K., Cretser, G. A., Lombardo, B., & Mathis, S. (1983). Fer cryin' out loud—There is a sex difference. *Sex Roles: A Journal of Research, 9*, 987–995.

Nelson, J. K. (2005). *Seeing through tears: Crying and attachment.* New York, NY: Routledge.

Owens, C. (2005). Moved to tears: Technical considerations and dilemmas encountered in working with a 13-year-old boy with acquired quadriplegia. *Journal of Child Psychotherapy, 31,* 284–302.

Pope, K. S., Tabachnick, B. G., & Keith-Spiegel, P. (1987). Ethics of practice: The beliefs and behaviors of psychologists as therapists. *American Psychologist, 42*, 993–1006.

Robinson, N., Hill, C. E., & Kivlighan, D. M. (2015). Crying as communication in psychotherapy: The influence of client and therapist attachment dimensions and client attachment to therapist on amount and type of crying. *Journal of Counseling Psychology, 62*(3), 379–392.

Searles, H. F. (1955). The informational value of the supervisor's emotional experiences. *Psychiatry: Journal for the Study of Interpersonal Processes, 18*, 135–146.

't Lam, C., & Vingerhoets, A. J. J. M. (2016). De tranen van de therapeut. [The tears of the therapist.] *De Psycholoog, 7,* 10–20.

Tracey, T. G., Bludworth, J., & Glidden-Tracey, C. E. (2011). Are there parallel processes in psychotherapy supervision? An empirical examination. *Psychotherapy, 49,* 330–343.

Tritt, A., Kelly, J., & Waller, G. (2015). Patients' experiences of clinicians' crying during psychotherapy for eating disorders. *Psychotherapy, 52*(3), 373–380.

Tsai, M., Kohlenberg, R. J., Kanter, J., Kohlenberg, B., Follette, W., & Callaghan, G. (2008). *A guide to functional analytic psychotherapy: Awareness, courage, love and behaviorism.* New York, NY: Springer.

Vingerhoets, A. J. J. M., & Bylsma, L. M. (2015). The riddle of human emotional crying: A challenge for emotion researchers. *Emotion Review,* 1–11.

Watson, A. (2015). *When therapists cry: Client's experience of witnessing therapist's tears. An interpretative phenomenological analysis.* Unpublished Honours dissertation. University of East London, London.

INDEX

abandonment: abuse and 134–135; child psychotherapy 175, 178; end-of-life therapy 148; fear of 48, 169; psychoanalysis 96; trauma survivors 138
abstinence 90, 91, 96
abuse 102–103, 131–140; caregiver tears 34; child psychotherapy 170, 171; compassion-focused therapy 109, 110, 111; emotional 188; *see also* trauma
Adams-Silvan, A. 145, 146
adolescents 35–36, 166–167, 169
affect matching 105, 109, 112
affect regulation 44, 46, 49, 50, 55, 86, 111–112; *see also* emotions
affective permeability 91–92
affective tone 169
affiliative emotions 104, 105, 106–107
age of therapist 29–30
aggression 14, 17, 95, 97, 193
agreeableness 31
Ainsworth, M. 46
alcohol abuse 134, 135, 137
Alexander, T. 16
altruism 9
Ancient Greeks 117
anger 10, 27, 102–103, 136–138, 171
anxiety 15, 47, 48–49, 109, 110; cancer and 144, 145, 146; child psychotherapy 170, 171; men 156; pregnant and postpartum patients 183, 185, 186–187, 188–189, 193; stranger 9; trauma recovery work 133
anxious attachment 207
attachment 11, 13, 32–33, 43–56, 74, 112; "attachment figures" 16; attachment style 46, 50–51, 207; compassion-focused therapy 104; crying as attachment behavior 9, 17, 207; crying as connection 52–53; evolutionary perspective 106, 107; pregnant and postpartum patients 194, 195; stages of grief 45–46, 48–50; therapeutic attachment bond 16, 47–48, 51–52
Atwood, G. 47
Augustine 125
authenticity 36, 93, 112, 215; child psychotherapy 166; end-of-life therapy 152; existential psychotherapy 118, 119, 120–121; psychodynamic theory 179; therapeutic immediacy 83, 84
avoidant attachment 207

Barbalet, J. 120, 126n6
Bartley, T. 146
"being-in-the-world" 117
"being-with" 121
Bekker, M. H. J. 11
bereavement 10, 45; child psychotherapy 170; therapists 53, 55; trauma recovery work 138–139, 140; *see also* death; grief; loss
Bering, J. M. 108
Big Five personality traits 31–32
Binder, J. L. 77
Bloomgarden, A. 59–72
Blume-Marcovici, A. 1–3, 23–39, 199–218
borderline personality disorder 16
Bowlby, J. 13, 33, 44, 45, 46
"boy code" 159, 162
brain 106
Brandell, J. R. 165–181
Bromberg, P. 93

INDEX

Brownlie, M. R. 24, 27, 32
Bruder, M. 12
Buddhism 104, 108
Bylsma, L. M. 7–22

Canada, A. L. 145
cancer 143, 144–150
Capps Umphlet, K. L. 73–88
caregiver tears 33, 34, 36
caregiving 33, 44–47, 55–56, 207; attachment style 46, 50–51; crying as connection 52–53; evolutionary psychology 106; stages of grief 45–46, 48, 49; termination of treatment 54
catharsis 11–12, 119
change 74, 76, 77, 85, 86, 112
chemotherapy 149
children: abusive childhoods 133–140; child psychotherapy 165–179; developmental changes 8–9; infanticide 191–193; termination of treatment 53–54; *see also* infants
classical psychoanalysis 92–93, 96
client-centered perspective 214, 215
clinical experience 28–30
cognition 117–118, 124
cognitive-behavioral therapy (CBT) 28, 145, 203
Cole, A. B. 146, 148
comfort 27, 84
communication 1, 93; child psychotherapy 167; non-verbal 68, 169–170; supervision 205
Community Connections 132–133
compassion 9, 104, 112, 134–135, 138; evolutionary perspective 106, 107–108; pregnant and postpartum patients 184, 185, 186, 188, 192, 195, 196; therapy with men 156
compassion-focused therapy (CFT) 101–112
confidentiality 67
Cornelius, R. R. 12
Counselman, E. F. 143–153
countertransference 47, 90–91, 92, 98; child psychotherapy 166, 171–172, 176–177, 179, 180n3; terminal illness 146
courage 36, 69, 112, 137, 183

crying 1–3, 7–17; antecedents and context of 10–11; attachment/caregiving perspective 43–56; child psychotherapy 166, 170–172, 175, 177–178, 179; clinical experience 28–30; compassion-focused therapy 102–103, 107, 108–112; developmental aspects 8–9; end-of-life therapy 147, 148, 149, 152; evolutionary perspective 8, 13–14, 107–108; existential psychotherapy 116, 119–125; frequency of 24–25, 37–38, 204, 207; functions of 7, 11–15; gender differences 10, 30–31, 207; health 15; impact on treatment 34–37, 38, 214; personality and 31–32; pregnant and postpartum patients 183–184, 185, 186, 187–196; psychoanalysis 89–90, 92, 93–98; reasons for 32–34; research on therapist crying 23–38; as self-disclosure 59–70; supervision 200–201; theoretical orientation 28; therapeutic immediacy 73–74, 78–86; therapy context 16–17; therapy with men 158–160, 161; training exercises 205–216; trauma recovery work 133–140
curiosity 2, 70

Darwin, Charles 8
Davies, J. M. 94
Davis, W. N. 183–197
death 146, 147, 148, 150–151; *see also* bereavement
defenses 77, 80, 146, 167, 170, 201
demeanor 28, 32, 35, 92
depression 13, 15, 199; attachment/caregiving perspective 49; cancer and 144, 145; child psychotherapy 170, 171; infanticide 192–193; postpartum 183, 185, 186–187, 188, 194; termination of therapy 178; trauma recovery work 133
despair 45–46, 49, 78; abused women 137; child psychotherapy 171; pregnant and postpartum patients 185, 186, 194; terminal illness 146; termination of therapy 178
detachment 45–46, 49–50
dignity 103–104
disappointment 10, 78

INDEX

discomfort 2, 27, 36, 47, 204
discussion of crying 37, 38, 179, 205, 214–215
dismissing attachment 11, 46, 51
disorganized attachment 46
dissociation 93, 97
divorce 156, 157, 170
dreams 168
drug use 115, 134, 137, 138, 139
Duberstein, P. R. 144
Dylan, Bob 136
dynamic child psychotherapy 166–170

eating disorders 25, 67
egocentrism 9
Ehrenberg, D. B. 94
emotional equilibrium 98
emotional expression 36, 37, 73–74, 80, 83–84; compassion-focused therapy 105; functional analytic psychotherapy 203; inhibition of 76–77; men 31, 156, 203; psychoanalysis 96, 98
emotional intelligence 112
emotions 10, 26–27, 107–108, 201; affiliative 104, 105, 106–107; cancer and 144–145; child psychotherapy 171, 172; compassion-focused therapy 104, 105, 109, 110, 111; end-of-life therapy 151; men 155, 156, 157, 159, 161, 162; mentalization 180n2; mixed 204–205; self-disclosure 61, 63, 66, 68–69; suppression of 111, 215; therapeutic immediacy 75, 79–80; *see also* affect regulation
empathy 11, 16, 28, 112, 215; child development 9; child psychotherapy 172; compassion-focused therapy 105, 109, 110, 111; empathic tears 33–34, 49; evolutionary perspective 107–108; existential psychotherapy 120–121; pregnant and postpartum patients 185, 188; trauma recovery work 140
enactments 92–93, 95, 98, 177
end-of-life therapy 143–152
ethnic groups 204
evolutionary perspective 8, 13–14, 104, 105–108

existential psychotherapy 115–125
extraversion 11, 31

facial expressions 44, 61, 169
Fairbairn, R. 94
fantasies: child psychotherapy 167, 168, 169, 170; countertransference 177; psychoanalysis 90, 92, 93, 98
Fawzy, F. I. 145
Fawzy, N. W. 145
fear 10, 98, 102; child psychotherapy 171; men 156; pregnant and postpartum patients 193
Fineberg, H. 171
Freud, Anna 166, 177
Freud, Sigmund 90–91, 126n4
frustration 10, 78, 107, 185
functional analytic psychotherapy 203

Gelman, R. 171
gender 8, 16; discussion of crying in supervision 202–203, 204; emotional situations 11, 210; frequency of crying 10, 30–31, 207; gender of client and therapist 31, 211; reactions to crying 15; traditional male gender role norms 155, 159, 161, 162; *see also* men; women
genuineness 36, 127n14, 147, 172, 179
Giambrone, S. 108
Gilbert, P. 104, 111
Gill, M. 91
goals of therapy 61–62, 85
Gračanin, A. 7–22
gratitude 27, 73, 80, 82, 85
Greeks, Ancient 117
grief 47–48, 107, 204; acute grief reactions 53, 55; attachment style 51; child psychotherapy 171, 172; crying as connection 52–53; empathic tears 33–34; pregnant and postpartum patients 184, 185, 186, 188; stages of 45–46, 48–50; termination of therapy 85; therapeutic attachment bond 51–52; *see also* bereavement; loss
group differences in crying 11
group treatment 132–133, 138, 139

INDEX

guilt 37, 48–49, 54; child development 9; child psychotherapy 169; existential psychotherapy 126n11; infanticide 192–193
Guntrip, H. 94

Hanser, W. E. 12
Harney, P. 89–100
Harris, M. 131–141
Hasson, O. 13–14, 107
healing 23, 172, 178, 183
health 12, 15, 146
Heidegger, M. 117, 119–120, 121, 126n2
Heinmann, P. 91
helplessness 9, 10, 16, 151, 159
Herman, J. 132
Hess, J. A. 75
Hill, C. E. 16, 56, 75, 85
Hilsenroth, M. J. 73–88
Hoffman, I. 91, 94
Hoover Dempsey, K. V. 14
hopelessness 10, 78, 84–85, 175
humanity 1, 60, 110–111, 116, 120, 123, 140
hypotheses 61, 62

individual differences in crying 10–11
infanticide 191–193
infants: attachment/caregiving perspective 13, 43, 44, 45–46, 49; evolutionary perspective 8, 106, 107–108; stranger anxiety 9; *see also* children
insecure attachment 46, 51
internal working models 46
interpersonal boundaries 195
interpersonal effects of crying 13–15
interpersonal psychoanalysis 91, 93
intersubjectivity 1; attachment/caregiving perspective 47, 49, 55, 56; child psychotherapy 175, 178, 179; compassion 107
intimacy 68, 80, 95, 107, 161, 169, 195
intraindividual effects of crying 11–13
Ivey, G. 92–93

joy 27, 34, 107, 138–139, 196; *see also* positive emotions

Kardum, I. 13
Keith-Spiegel, P. 24
Keller, M. C. 15
Kelly, J. 24
Khademi, M. 23–39, 199–218
Kierkegaard, Søren 117
kinesic cues 169–170
Kivlighan, D. M. 16, 56
Klein, Melanie 166, 177
Kleinian psychoanalysis 92–93, 96, 97
Kohrman, R. 171, 180n3
Kübler-Ross, E. 145
Kuutmann, K. 73–88

listening 167–168, 179, 187
loss 9, 27, 44, 45–46, 47–48; abused women 134–135; child psychotherapy 170; crying as connection 52–53; empathic tears 33–34; psychoanalysis 96; stages of grief 48–50; termination of therapy 82–83, 85; *see also* bereavement; grief
love 7, 95, 136
Luborsky, L. 77

MacCormack, T. 146–147, 152
Mackie, A. 23–39
Marguiles, A. 94
Mark, R. E. 12
Mayotte-Blum, J. 73–88
McCullough, L. 75, 77
McGinley, P. 115–128
McWilliams, N. 94
meaning 117–118, 120, 122, 124, 125, 126n2
Meissner, W. W. 144–145, 146
melancholia 8
men: discussion of crying in supervision 202–203, 204; emotional situations 210; frequency of crying 10, 30–31, 207; gender of client and therapist 31, 211; therapy with 155–163; *see also* gender
mental health 15, 185–186, 193
mentalization 167, 180n2
Merleau-Ponty, M. 122
metaphors 156, 157, 167
mindfulness 104, 108, 109, 111–112, 146, 215

INDEX

Mitchell, S. 91–92
mood 12–13
mood disorders 15, 185, 186, 187, 193
Muran, J. C. 75
music 157, 158, 160
mutuality 1, 44, 47, 69

narcissistic personality disorder 16
negative arousal 44–45, 46, 47, 48
Nelson, J. K. 13, 24, 26, 43–57
Nesse, R. M. 15
neuroticism 11, 31
non-verbal communication 68, 169–170
normalization 204

object relations 169
openness 31, 92
otherness 119, 122, 125
Ovid 7
Owens, C. 200–201

pain 9, 48, 78, 107; cancer patients 145, 150; men 156; pregnant and postpartum patients 184; see also suffering
paralinguistic cues 169–170
parallel process 205
parents 9, 66; child psychotherapy 167, 169, 172; family of origin issues 78, 188–189; loss of 170
Parkinson, B. 12
Pendleton, K. 35–36
personality 11, 13, 15, 16, 31–32
perspective-taking 105, 107–108, 110; see also empathy
phenomenology 118, 120, 121, 122, 126n3
Piaget, Jean 168
Pinquart, M. 144
Plas, J. M. 14
play 167, 168, 169, 170, 173–174
pleasure, tears of 171
Pollin, I. 150
Pope, K. S. 24
positive emotions 10, 27, 30; see also joy
postpartum depression (PPD) 183, 185, 186–187, 188, 194
postpartum psychosis 191–193
Povinelli, D. J. 108

powerlessness 9, 10, 27, 133, 137, 175
pregnant and postpartum patients 183–196
preoccupied attachment 46, 51
primary process 167, 168, 170, 173–174
professionalism 23, 35, 152
projective identification 91, 97, 201
protest 45, 48–49, 51–52, 54
proud-parent tears 33, 34
psychoanalysis 89–98, 145, 171–172
psychodynamic approaches 11, 28, 29, 77–78, 179, 203
psychoeducation 194–195
psychosis, postpartum 191–193
psychosocial development 169

Rabinowitz, F. E. 155–163
rape 134, 137
rapport 16, 36, 205
reactions to crying 14–15
regret about crying 27, 29
rejection 110, 169
relational psychoanalysis 91–92, 93, 96, 171–172
relationships 11, 74; case examples 77, 78, 84; compassion 108; ending 97; existential psychotherapy 123; reactions to crying 15; therapeutic immediacy 75
remorse about crying 27
Renik, O. 98
resilience 111, 112
resistance 77, 156
responsibility 118
retirement 52, 54–55
Richman, J. 146
Robinson, N. 16, 56
role reversal 36, 37, 172
Rottenberg, J. 13

Saakvitne, K. 94
sadness 10, 27, 47, 133; abused women 138; child psychotherapy 171; compassion-focused therapy 102–103, 109–110; men 156, 159, 162; mixed emotions 204; pregnant and postpartum patients 185, 188, 189; therapeutic immediacy 78, 80, 85
Safran, J. D. 75

Saigyō, S. 119
Sandler, J. 91
Sartre, Jean-Paul 117, 124
schizophrenia 15, 174
Schraufnagel, K. E. 199–218
secure attachment 46, 50–51, 112, 207
self 93, 119, 120, 168, 169
self-acceptance 162
self-awareness 56, 85, 93, 106
self-care 195
self-comfort 12
self-compassion 95–96, 106, 109, 110, 111
self-control 95
self-criticism 109, 110, 111, 188, 189
self-disclosure 59–70; case examples 64–68; child psychotherapy 166, 176, 177; client preferences 63–64; compassion-focused therapy 109; end-of-life therapy 143, 147, 151, 152; existential psychotherapy 121; intentional or unintentional 61; supervision 204; therapeutic 61–63
self-reflection 67, 179, 191, 206
self-sacrifice 9
sentimentality, tears of 9
separation 8, 45–46, 54, 96
shame 2, 95, 109, 204; child psychotherapy 171; infanticidal mothers 191, 192; men 156, 162; pregnant and postpartum patients 184, 186, 193, 194–195, 196
Shyamalan, M. N. 166, 178
Silberstein, L. R. 101–113
Šimić, M. 13
Simons, G. 12
The Sixth Sense (film) 165–166, 172–179
Slochower, J. 94
social bonding 14, 17
social support 144
societal pain 9
"species-preservative" system 106
Spidell, K. 43
Spiegel, D. 145
stage of therapy 26, 51–52
stillbirth 186, 187, 188–189
Stolberg, R. A. 23–39, 199–218
Stolorow, R. 47
stranger anxiety 9
strategies 62

stress 15, 77, 185
Strupp, H. H. 77
suffering 23, 124–125, 134, 140; children's sympathy 9; compassion-focused therapy 104, 105, 108, 109–111; Darwin 8; pregnant and postpartum patients 184, 194; ritual weeping 14; *see also* pain
suicidality 50, 95, 134, 199–200, 201
suicide 192, 194
supervision 53, 199–216
supervisory alliance 203–204
surveys 2, 12, 14, 24–27, 37, 202, 204
sympathy 17, 105

't Lam, C. 23–39, 202
Tabachnick, B. G. 24
taboo 2, 95, 162, 186
Ter Bogt, T. F. M. 12
terminal illness 143–152
termination of therapy 34, 53–54, 73–74, 96–98; forced 204; as microtrauma 178; therapeutic immediacy 75, 80–83, 85
Thalenberg, E. 43
theory of mind 9
therapeutic alliance 2, 207; child psychotherapy 168, 174; compassion-focused therapy 104, 112; men 162
therapeutic immediacy 73–86
therapeutic relationship: adaptive relating 77; attachment/caregiving perspective 47–48, 51–52, 56; compassion-focused therapy 104, 109; end-of-life therapy 147; functional analytic psychotherapy 203; impact of crying on 36; pregnant and postpartum patients 185, 187; psychoanalysis 93; self-disclosure 60, 64, 66, 68, 70; termination of therapy 80, 83, 85; therapeutic immediacy 74–75, 86
Tirch, D. 101–113
training 125, 202, 203, 205–216
transference 90–91, 92
transparency 63–64, 65, 121, 123, 125
trauma 55, 109, 204; caregiver tears 34; child psychotherapy 171, 172; childbirth-related 193; trauma recovery work 132–140; *see also* abuse
Treadway, D. 61–62

treatment, types of 25–26
Tritt, A. 24, 25, 30, 32, 35
triumph, tears of 34, 138–139
trust 67–68, 80, 96, 184, 195

Unit, B. 107

values 117, 123, 124
Van der Lowe, I. 12
Van Tol, A. J. M. 12
Vingerhoets, A. J. J. M. 7–22, 24–25, 34, 36, 202
violence 134, 136–137, 139
visual cues 169–170
vocalization 8, 9
vulnerability 2, 60; children 9; evolutionary perspective 107; men 159, 161; new parents 194–195; psychoanalysis 92, 97; self-disclosure 63, 66, 68, 69; therapeutic immediacy 80; working with cancer patients 146

Wachtel, P. L. 75, 77
Waldman, J. L. 29, 31, 34
Waller, G. 24
Wang, S. 106
warmth 27, 147, 204
Watson, A. 35, 37
Weiss, S. 171
Wilber, K. 145, 150
witnessing 140, 186
women: acceptability of female tears 162; cancer patients 145; discussion of crying in supervision 202–203; emotional situations 11, 210; frequency of crying 10, 30–31, 207; gender of client and therapist 31, 211; pregnant and postpartum patients 183–196; trauma recovery work 132–140; *see also* gender

Yalom, I. 69

Zupčić, M. 13

Taylor & Francis eBooks

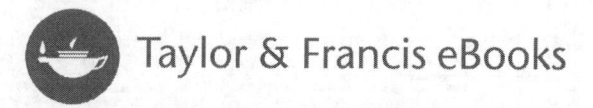

Helping you to choose the right eBooks for your Library

Add Routledge titles to your library's digital collection today. Taylor and Francis ebooks contains over 50,000 titles in the Humanities, Social Sciences, Behavioural Sciences, Built Environment and Law.

Choose from a range of subject packages or create your own!

Benefits for you
- Free MARC records
- COUNTER-compliant usage statistics
- Flexible purchase and pricing options
- All titles DRM-free.

Benefits for your user
- Off-site, anytime access via Athens or referring URL
- Print or copy pages or chapters
- Full content search
- Bookmark, highlight and annotate text
- Access to thousands of pages of quality research at the click of a button.

REQUEST YOUR FREE INSTITUTIONAL TRIAL TODAY

Free Trials Available
We offer free trials to qualifying academic, corporate and government customers.

eCollections – Choose from over 30 subject eCollections, including:

Archaeology	Language Learning
Architecture	Law
Asian Studies	Literature
Business & Management	Media & Communication
Classical Studies	Middle East Studies
Construction	Music
Creative & Media Arts	Philosophy
Criminology & Criminal Justice	Planning
Economics	Politics
Education	Psychology & Mental Health
Energy	Religion
Engineering	Security
English Language & Linguistics	Social Work
Environment & Sustainability	Sociology
Geography	Sport
Health Studies	Theatre & Performance
History	Tourism, Hospitality & Events

For more information, pricing enquiries or to order a free trial, please contact your local sales team: **www.tandfebooks.com/page/sales**

Routledge
Taylor & Francis Group

The home of Routledge books

www.tandfebooks.com